Walking

and Light Running

Dr. Klaus Bös
In cooperation with Sylvie Hinderberger
and Susanne Tittlbach

BARNES
& NOBLE
NEW YORK

This 2006 edition published by Barnes & Noble, Inc., by arrangement with GRÄFE UND UNZER VERLAG GmbH, Munich

Picture credits:
Peter von Felbert (Cover, p. 11, 128); Leonhard Lenz (Outdoor-Fotos People); Marcel Weber (Indoor-Fotos People, Stills)

Additional photos:
Baby-Walz: p. 116. Corbis: p. 44, 112. Excel: p. 78. GU: p. 64 (B. Büchner); 2 l., 6, 62 (A. Hosch); 30, back cover inside (M. Jahreiß); 115 (A. Peisl); 86 (T. Roch); 43, 68, 69 (R. Schmitz); 54 (M. Wagenhan). Jump: p. 4, 15 (M. Sandkühler); 70, 117, 120 (K. Vey). Zefa: p. 61.

Illustrations:
Detlef Seidensticker

Production:
bookwise Medienproduktion GmbH, Munich

Translation:
Trahern Gemmell

Important notice
The author and publisher have made every effort to ensure the information provided in this book conforms to national health and fitness standards and that the exercises are suitable for healthy individuals. It is not meant to replace the advice of a physician. Each reader is asked to make a personal decision as to which exercises are appropriate and how closely they want to follow the advice in this book. Neither the author nor publisher can assume responsibility for any injury, loss or harm resulting from the practices offered in this book.

ISBN (13): 978-0-7607-8494-5
ISBN (10): 0-7607-8494-9

Printed and bound in China

1 3 5 7 9 10 8 6 4 2

Foreword

These days I encounter speed walkers everywhere: in the park, on the street, in group and on their own. Millions of people now speed walk, part of them in organized walking groups and walking meets hosted by clubs or fitness studios – most, however, go solo.
Speed walking has its roots in the USA and in the long tradition of sport-oriented hiking in Germany. Nordic walking, or walking with special poles, has long been known in Scandinavia as a summer variant of cross-country skiing. I have been promoting this health- and sport-oriented activity in Germany for 15 years now, and in the last ten years speed walking has slowly developed into a national sport – for good reason!
This light sport is suitable for almost all people, regardless of whether they have previous athletic experience or not. In contrast to running there is no high-speed phase – this is why it is so easy on the joints and well-suited for beginners, seniors, and people who are overweight. But I recommend speed walking also for fitness enthusiasts and the athletically experienced. You too will find demanding variants to speed walking or Nordic walking, with which you can really put yourself to the challenge.
Sports science defines speed walking as "athletic and health-oriented walking with a heart rate of 120 to 140 beats per minute and a speed between 4 and 5.5 miles per hour". Because speed walking comes very close to the human body's natural motion patterns, it is easily learned and has a positive effect on one's health. It also helps you on the way to achieving your dream figure and greater fitness. So what more could you want? Step right into your own personal speed walking program! The book in your hands will help you with this and give you all you need to know about technique, equipment, and training plans.

Dr. Klaus Bös

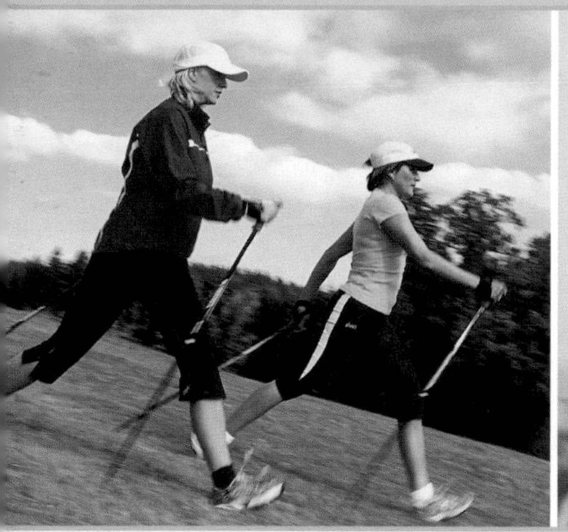

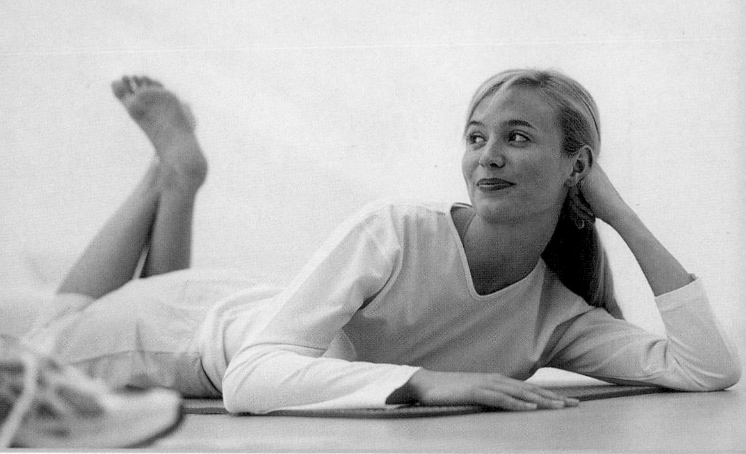

CONTENTS

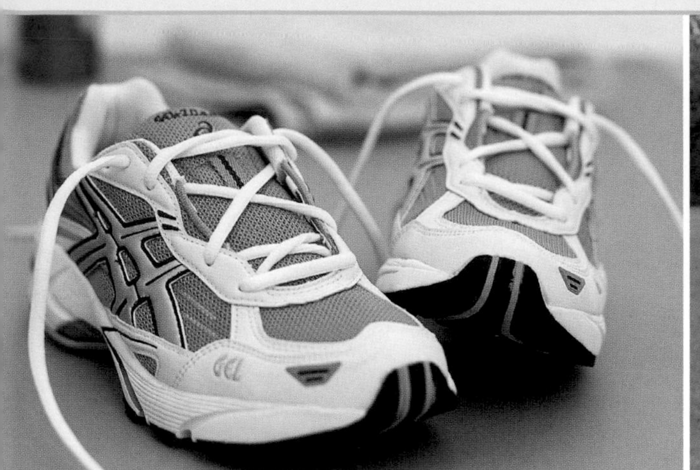

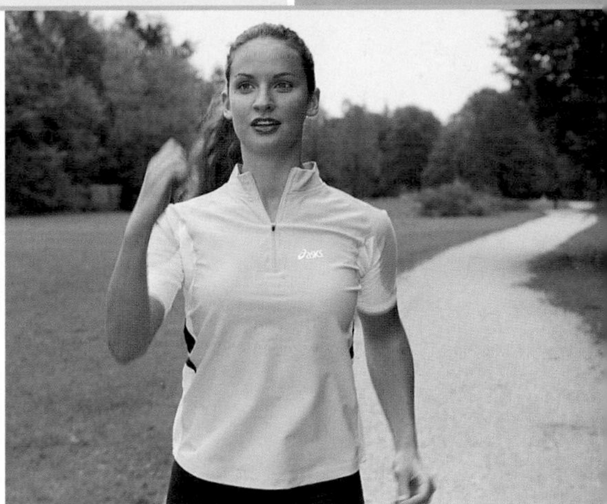

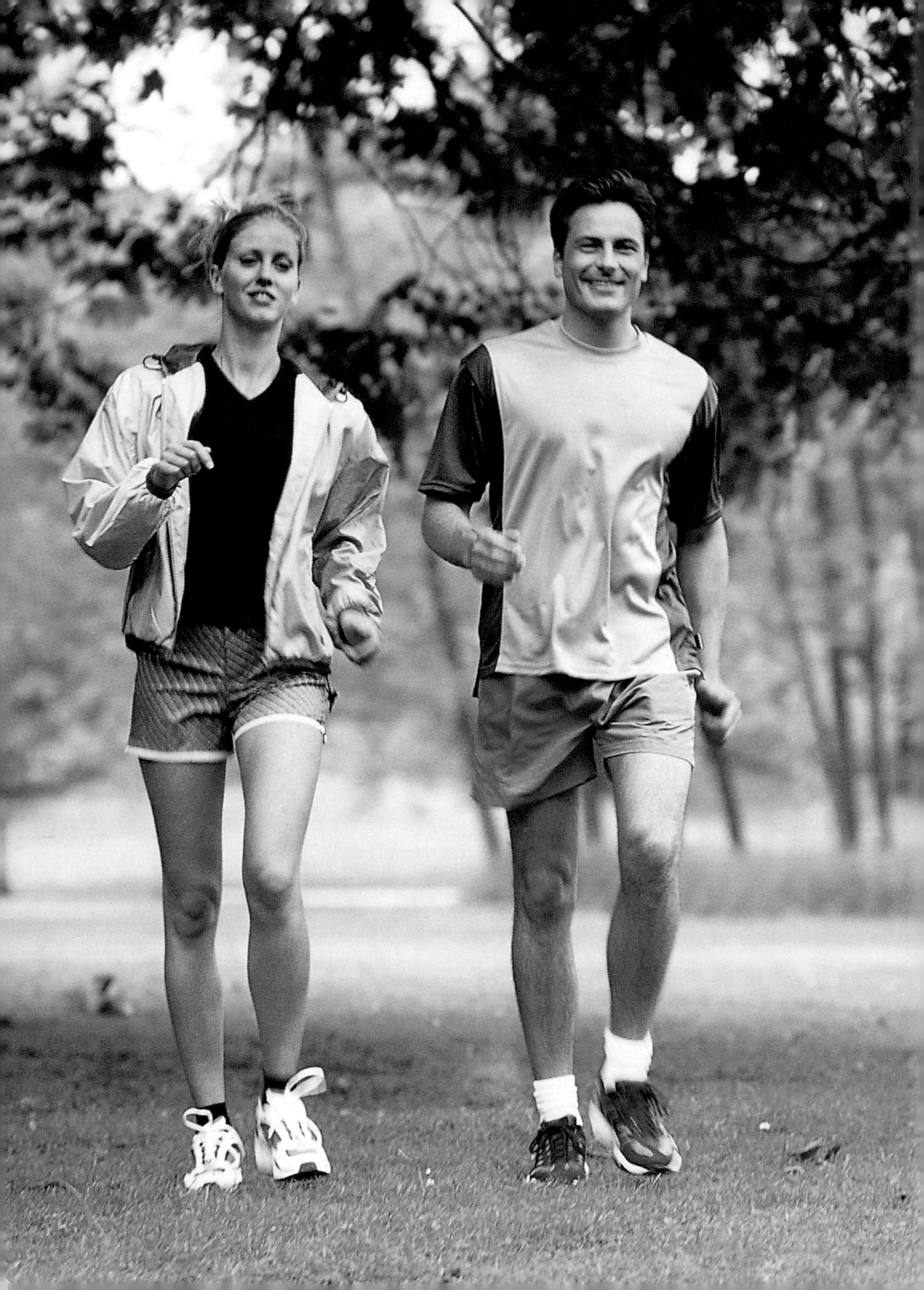

Healthy, skinny, and relaxed

You want to do more for your health and fitness and also lose a few pounds while you're at it? Forget sweat-drenching action and get speed walking instead. This light endurance training will ensure that you are in top shape regardless of whether you're old or young, thin or overweight, beginner or athlete – speed walking is right for everyone!

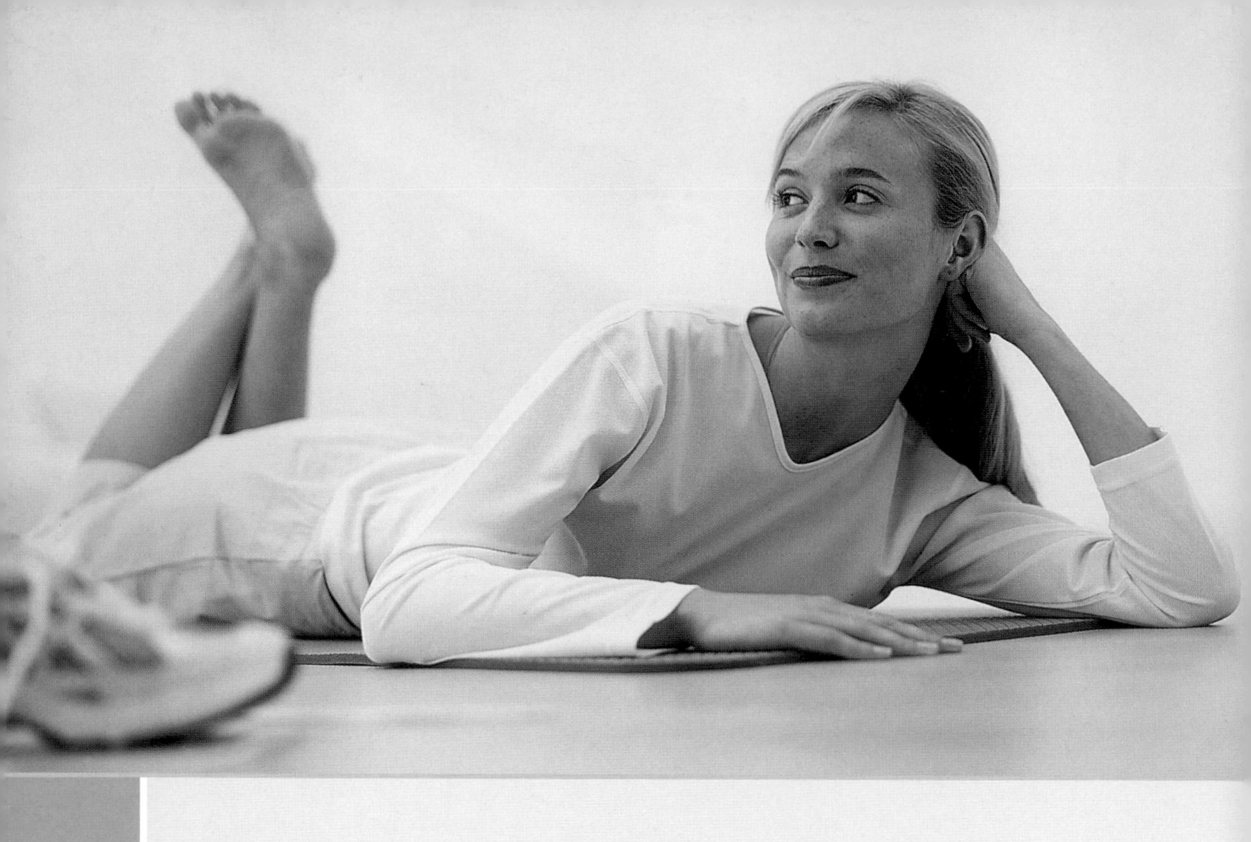

Walk yourself fit!

Speed walking is booming – and for good reason! Don't let the name fool you: speed walking does not mean merely strolling through the outdoors. When speed walking, you hold yourself decidedly upright and take quick steps, during which your arms angle and swing along at a rhythmic rate. With each step you roll your foot consciously from heel to ball and actively push it away from the ground. With the proper technique speed walking becomes the optimal full-body sport: through the quick, but not overly long, steps and the powerful ankle joint and calf activity you train both legs and your backside. By involving the arms you also simultaneously strengthen your back, shoulder, and arm muscles. In contrast to the competitive sport "walking" with its extreme hip rotations, speed, and competition are not what really count with speed walking, but rather fun, fitness, and health.

All good reasons for speed walking

100 years ago people still had to travel an average of 30 miles a day on foot to meet everyday demands. Today only ten percent of the population has a career which is also physically demanding. While our ancestors often burned more calories in a day than they could consume, the energy balance is swinging the other way in our modern society.

In contrast to declining physical career demands, however, our mental and spiritual burden continually increases. Already half of the working population complains of stress and suffers from psychological imbalance, irritability, sleep disorders, and lack of exercise. One of the best means to fight these "damages to civilization" is called speed walking. With speed walking you are not only doing good things for your health and figure but you also learn how to better cope with stress. The result: you feel better all around.

Fit through speed walking

If you're fit, you can take long breaths and not get winded so quickly. For instance, while sprinting for the morning bus, you might take quick, shallow breaths which will not disperse oxygen efficiently throughout your body, and in particular your muscles. The oxygen will be exhaled without being put to use.

Healthy through speed walking

It is still fiercely disputed whether sports are a prerequisite for a long and healthy life. It is, however, indisputable that physical activity significantly improves one's health. It was determined in a long-term study that the risk of heart attack is reduced by about 25 percent if you burn an additional 800 to 1,000 calories a week through physical/athletic activity. To achieve this increased energy consumption you have to merely spend two hours a week engaged in moderate endurance sports.

But lack of time is a beloved argument when it comes to neglecting athletic activity. For this reason, sports can take on a compensating function when career, family, and household pull the time corset tighter and tighter. Research has shown that sports help to cope with the burdens of the everyday.
In contrast to non-athletes, the athletically active displayed decidedly better health conditions. While no negative health effects from career pressures were perceived in the case of the athletically active, doctors classed non-athletes as less healthy even under equal career pressures.

INFO

BE A WINNER WITH SPEED WALKING

- Your circulatory system is significantly stabilized.
- Your metabolism works considerably more efficiently.
- Your motion and support system becomes capable of more.
- Your immune system is strengthened.
- Your psyche is positively influenced.
- Your self-image is strengthened.
- You stay young, attractive, and mobile longer.
- You stay (or become) thin.
- You reduce stress.

Women and speed walking

For women speed walking offers further advantages. It protects against osteoporosis for one. If you walk regularly, bone development and disintegration remain in balance longer – meaning the skeletal system becomes more stable. At the same time, bones are increasingly supplied with minerals by the light tensile and pressure loads which speed walking affords. Speed walking works to prevent cellulite by strengthening your muscles, especially those in your legs and backside. The connective tissue becomes firmer and those bothersome dimples get smaller or even disappear altogether. There is also nothing to prevent a woman from speed walking during her period. Today few women believe they have to go easy on themselves physically during their period. Indeed they can be extremely athletic on these days.

As many as 80 percent of all women suffer from premenstrual syndrome (PMS) in the days leading up to their period, and from symptoms such as breast tension, abdominal pains, headaches, migraines, or general irritability. The physical and emotional symptoms are supposed to be triggered chiefly by hormonal swings within the female cycle as well as by an imbalance in certain neurotransmitters. But individual factors such as the wrong foods, stress, and insufficient physical fitness can also contribute to such complaints. A light endurance training such as speed walking can ease these problems. Besides exercise and fresh air, the cramp-preventing nature of speed walking helps the most. Not only that but the hormones released by exercise also improve one's mood.

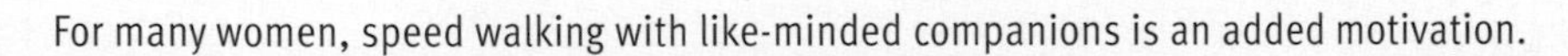

For many women, speed walking with like-minded companions is an added motivation.

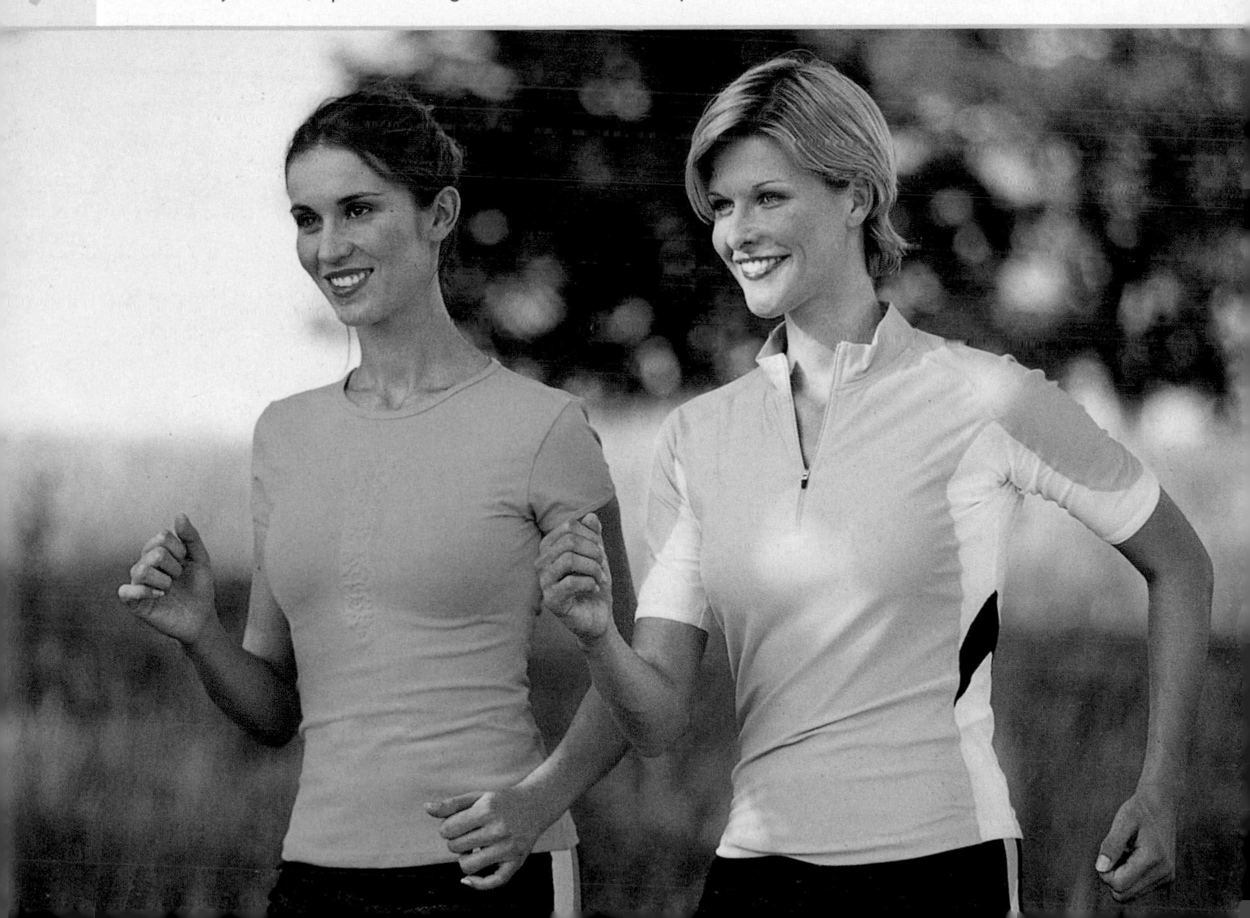

Speed walking during pregnancy

Speed walking is especially suitable as a light form of training during pregnancy. The heart pumps more blood through the circulatory system and thus ensures that mother and child are optimally provided with oxygen. Decisive for this positive effect, however, is not that you go full steam every now and again but rather that you train lightly on a regular basis, ideally two to three times a week. Also, this exercise improves body posture, which prevents back pain.

A further plus: speed walking prevents classic pregnancy complaints such as varicose veins and calf cramps. It even helps prevent hormonally triggered mood swings during pregnancy, because the endorphins released during speed walking create positive emotions.

Additionally, the babies of physically active mothers are especially vivacious after birth. So, you can begin speed walking even during pregnancy.

A special training guide for mothers and pregnant women can be found on page 112. But be careful: the distensibility of tendons and ligaments increases during pregnancy, so that joints are especially at risk. Definitely make sure you have the proper speed walking technique and good shoes. You should also exercise on the most level terrain possible.

Regular speed walking also brings pleasing results to the scale.

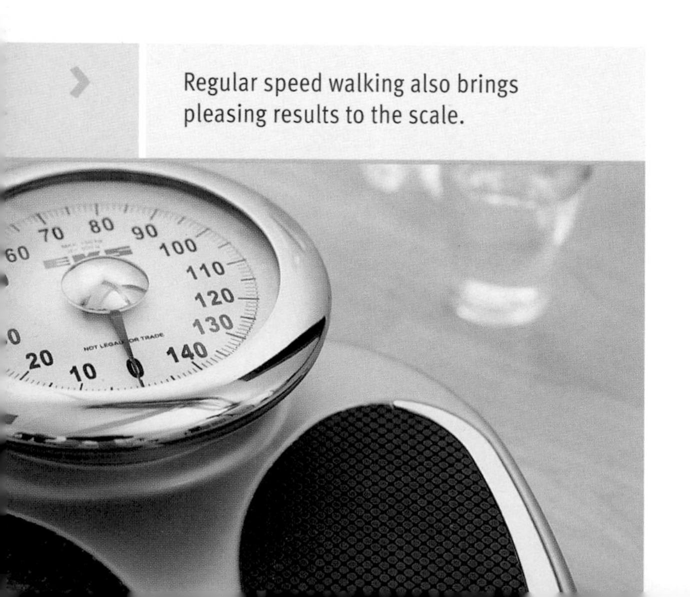

Losing weight with speed walking

Good news for everyone who wants to finally lose weight for the long term: the pounds roll away as well during speed walking! It isn't a matter of going as fast as possible. What's important is that you speed walk regularly and in the aerobic range, that is, with an oxygen surplus (see page 30). This is

HOW MANY CALORIES DO YOU BURN?

Sports science has developed a method in the past few years by which one can determine individual energy consumption during various activities with relative precision. The number of metabolic units (METS) is determined for each activity. This is a measure of oxygen intake that can be converted into a measure of energy consumption. According to this, 1 MET equals exactly 1 kcal per kilogram of body weight per hour, thus the basal metabolic rate. That sounds more complicated than it is:

Physical activity type (mean intensity)	**Personal calorie consumption** (metabolic unit per hour)
watching television, reading	1 MET x body weight in kg
kissing, laughing	2 METS x body weight in kg
bowling	3 METS x body weight in kg
bicycling	4 METS x body weight in kg
gardening (raking, etc.)	4 METS x body weight in kg
gymnastics	4 METS x body weight in kg
strolling	4 METS x body weight in kg
ergometric training	5 METS x body weight in kg
speed walking	5 METS x body weight in kg
mountain hiking	6 METS x body weight in kg
jogging, cross-country skiing	7 METS x body weight in kg
inline skating	7 METS x body weight in kg

As a rule of thumb: multiply the number of METS by your body weight in kilograms (1 kg = 2,204 lbs) and you will get the number of calories you consume in one hour. **Example:** A woman weighing 60 kg (132 lbs) consumes 5 METS 60 kg = 300 calories during speed walking. A woman weighing 90 kg consumes in contrast 5 METS 90 kg (198 lbs) = 450 calories. Because with each step a greater mass must be moved, the calorie consumption is proportionally higher with a higher starting weight. Two to three hours of speed walking per week thus fulfill the necessary health criterium of 800 to 1,000 additional calories per week.

when your body burns the most calories and the capacity for weight loss is highest. The body's basal metabolic weight increases simultaneously in this manner. You consume more energy – not only during speed walking but the whole day.

Feeling good all-around

Speed walking doesn't just positively affect our fitness and physical health but our psyche as well. Just one hour of speed walking a week can noticeably improve our well-being. Exercise in the outdoors helps to better process stress and problems, both everyday and career-related, because your metabolism is activated during speed walking and the creativity hormone ACTH is released. Concentration and attention span are also noticeably increased with fresh air. Whoever is looking to tune out, then, should choose paths on which there are no distractions from traffic, noise, or exhaust but where recuperation in open nature is guaranteed. If you speed walk you more consciously perceive your body and ensure that it functions better. The interplay of muscles, good circulation, and the recognition of your own physical capacity have a positive influence on self-image and your perception of self-worth.
Another positive side effect of speed walking should not be forgotten at this juncture: speed walking makes you attractive! Because each breath while walking brings in up to eight times more oxygen, cell regeneration is powerfully accelerated and skin is toned. The lost pounds and your body's contours, which firm up when you strengthen your muscles, do something for your self-image!

TIP

GOOD AMUSEMENT!

If you don't like to speed walk alone, seek out those with similar interests with whom you can talk underway. As long as you can converse while walking, that is a reliable sign that you're walking in the aerobic range. If you don't find a speed walking partner, you can also amuse yourself with music or an audio book.

Walking instead of running

Scientific studies have proven that often the over-exertion during runnig is so high that the training actually has rather a negative effect

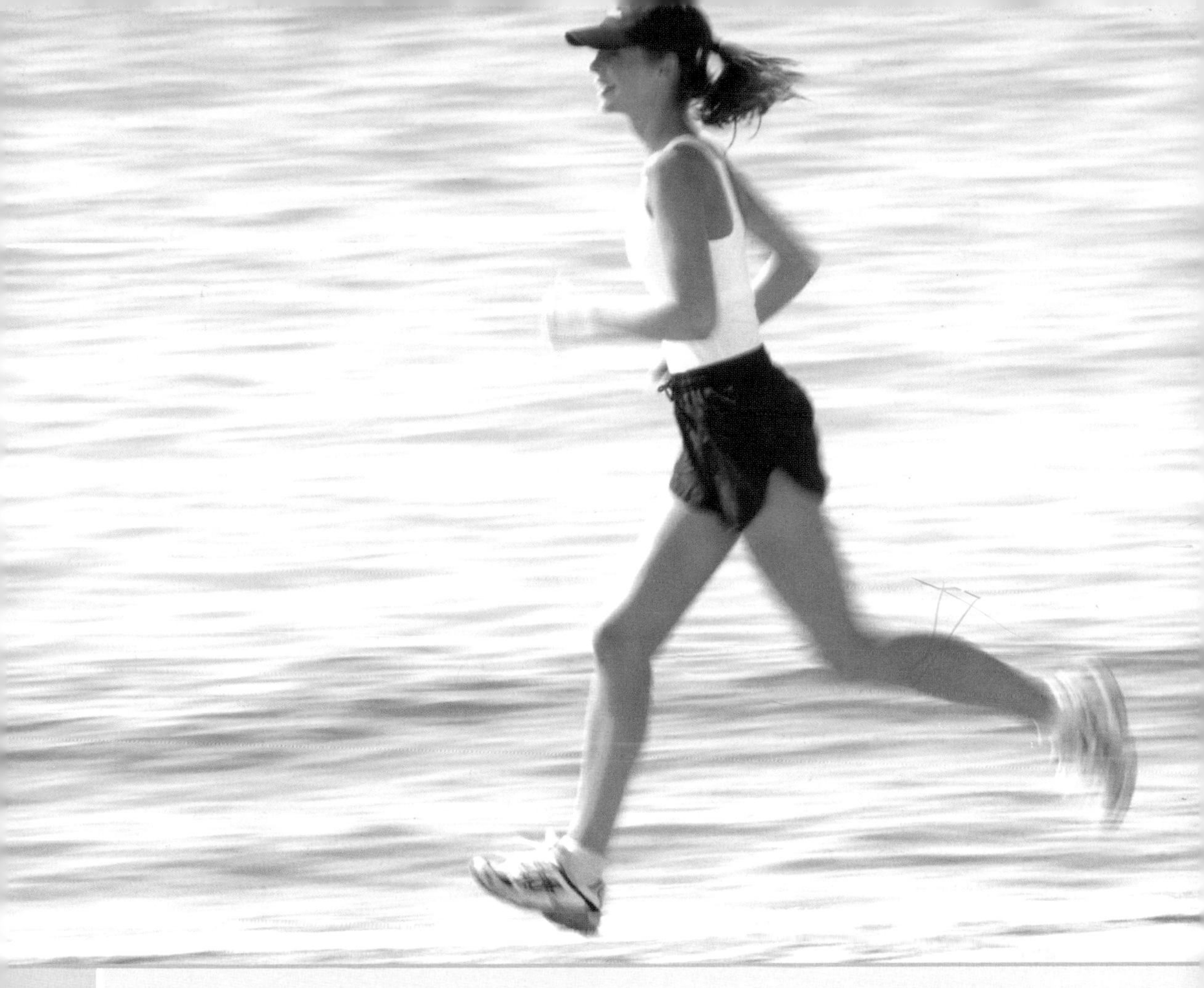

Unlike speed walking, running has a short high-speed phase that can burden the joints.

on the health and the body's movement apparatus. Many orthopedists have also been complaining for years that more overburdening damages occur to the ankle, knee, and hip joints through over-exertive running.
The danger of overload during speed walking is, on the contrary, extremely low. Joints, tendons, ligaments, and vertebrae are significantly less burdened than with other sports. In the case of jogging, for instance, the forces necessary for pushing off from the ground equal at least three times one's body weight.
With speed walking your joints only have to suspend a force equal to one or two times your body weight. The reason: in contrast to running there is no high-speed phase and one foot always remains in contact with the ground.

INFO

A COMPARISON OF SPEED WALKING AND RUNNING

Are you still undecided about whether you should speed walk or run?
Make the comparison yourself:

Speed walking	Running
No airborne phase, meaning less contact shock	Airborne phase, meaning higher contact shock
Minimal joint burden	Burden to joints is higher
Little training effect for the experienced	Positive training effect for the experienced as we
Adjustable training intensity	Risk of over-exertion
Suitable for almost everybody, also for people with health problems	Especially for young, experienced athletes of normal weight
Minimal risk of injury	Risk of injury higher than with speed walking

The risk of arthritis or other inflammatory joint disorders is also significantly less. As endurance training, speed walking is ideal for those out of practice, for overweight people, and even for those with orthopedic ailments because, with the proper technique, there is practically no risk of injury. Speed walking is counted as one of the soft endurance sports and is thus suitable for all age groups and every fitness level, the reason being that the intensity can be easily controlled even by beginners. Jogging offers an advantage mostly in the case that an athlete has already reached a certain level and feels under-challenged by speed walking.

Speed walking: Sport for the masses

The days of sweat-inducing fitness regimens are over. With speed walking you don't have to tire yourself out like with running. Because of this, it is easier to hold out for at least 30 minutes (the period of effectiveness for health) and to stay on the ball for a greater length of time.
So it's no wonder that speed walking speaks to a wide audience. Even those who feel they are not fit enough, too awkward, or too old for other sports

such as running or aerobics have little contact fear when it comes to speed walking. The reason is that it consists mostly of everyday cycles of motion and is thus easy for the inexperienced as well. Also, speed walking can be integrated into your daily routine without any problem. With the proper shoes you can speed walk at any time and any place. In contrast to other endurance sports such as swimming or inline skating you need no swimming pool and don't have to learn any difficult technique to speed walk. Instead, beginners and sport laggards need simply step through the door and speed walk away.

Risk check

Even though speed walking is counted as one of the low-risk sports, there are a few factors which make it a good idea to consult a doctor before training. If, for example, you've participated in no sports for more than two years, you should get the OK of your family doctor before beginning training. This is especially important if you:

- have had a heart attack or stroke,
- are aware of any heart murmur or arterial constriction,
- sense any chest pains (with or without a radiation through the left side of your body or shortness of breath),
- have circulatory disturbances (with or without pins and needles in the affected body parts),
- have high blood pressure,
- have highly pronounced varicose veins or a tendency for thrombosis,
- feel weight pains in your legs after walking no more than 300 feet,
- suffer from a chronic illness (for example, diabetes mellitus, rheumatism, or an arterial disorder),
- have joint complaints,
- have an acute infection (fever), feel unwell or weak,
- have experienced a lengthy hospital stay or were in the hospital the previous year,
- feel weak or dizzy when you walk fast,
- frequently feel extreme fatigue.

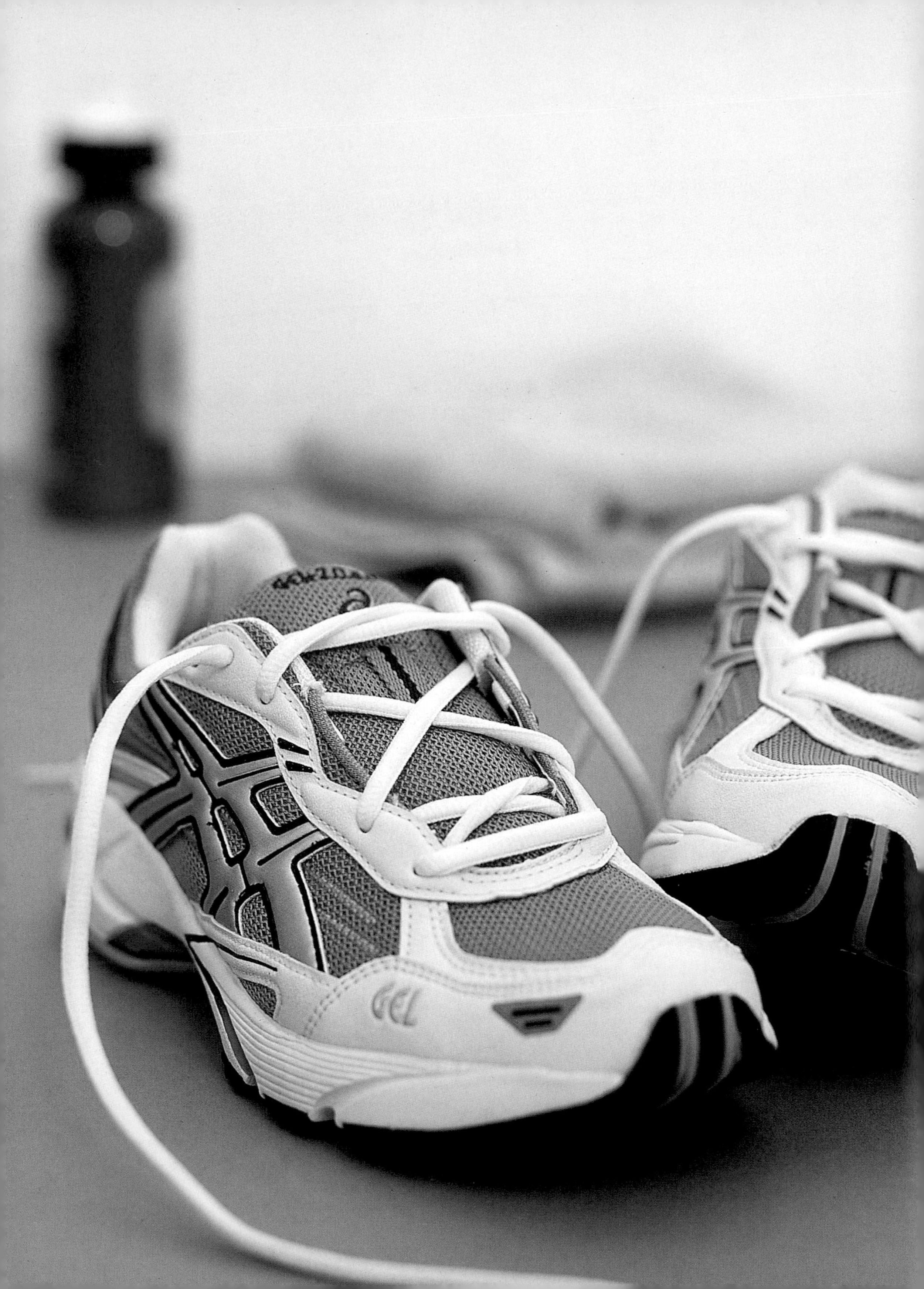
GEL

walking!

Have you decided to begin training? Nothing better than stepping into those speed walking shoes, then here you will learn everything you need to know – from the proper technique and warm-up to selecting the proper clothes and keeping the optimal diet. A stamina checkup and speed walking programs for every fitness level will then help you succeed.

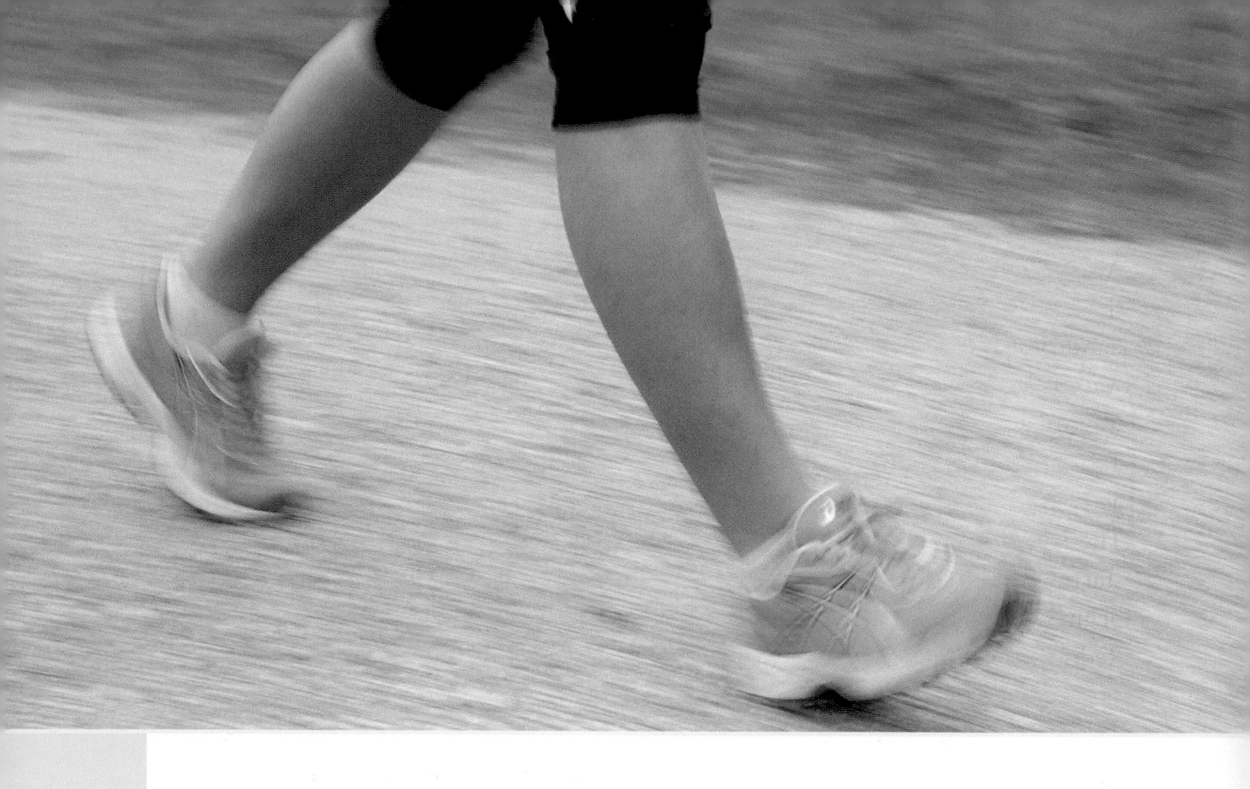

Stamina checkup

Even if walking is the ideal beginner's sport, you do need some conditioning before you start training. Here it's not so much a matter of speed. On the contrary, you should not walk too fast, espacially when you want to burn fat. The following endurance test was specially designed for speed walking and can be playfully integrated into your training program. For this you will need:

- Pen and paper to record your time and pulse,
- good running shoes (page 57),
- a stopwatch to determine your walking time in minutes and seconds, and to measure your pulse.

The walking test

- Choose a level route for the test of about one mile. Ride the route beforehand on a bicycle with an odometer. Alternatively, you can speed walk five laps on a sports field with a quarter-mile track.

- Avoid a cold start: To warm up before the test, walk 350–500 yards before hand. Slowly increase your speed and walk as fast as you can at the end. This way you get a feel for the proper tempo. Take a breather before you begin the actual test.
- Then let's get to it: Record the starting time with a stopwatch and begin walking as quickly as possible. Reduce your tempo, though, as soon as you begin running out of breath, because otherwise your pulse will rise too much.
- After you have speed walked a mile, stop the watch and record the minutes and seconds you needed for the stretch walked.
- Then measure your pulse. Feel the pulse on your wrist (page 29) and count the beats for 15 seconds. Record the number of beats before multiplying them by four to get the number per minute.

Assessing your walking time

Look over the chart on page 22 to see your fitness and endurance level. While doing this, make sure that your evaluation does not take into consideration age and capacity alone, but gender as well.
Women naturally have less muscle mass and less body weight than do men. Both determine heart volume, as does heart muscle size, i.e. the quantity of blood that can be pumped through your body with each heart beat. This in turn determines the maximum oxygen intake capacity as well as a person's maximum endurance level.

Your Personal Figure

First, find your age group on the chart. Three differing walking times are given for each age group: in the center are the times test walkers reach on average, left of this the somewhat worse, right the somewhat better.

Target Pulse Frequency

To evaluate your fitness level you need more than just the time. You also must put walking time into proportion with your pulse under strain, that is, the pulse you measure at the end of your test.
In contrast to differing fitness levels regarding endurance, men and women are evaluated equally when it comes to their pulse. Look again for your figure on the chart on page 23 in the appropriate age group.

CALCULATION OF WALKING TIME FOR THE WOMEN'S WALKING TEST

Walking time in minutes : seconds for women

age	below average min. : sec.	average min. : sec.	above average min. : sec.
20	>16:20	15:25–16:20	<15:25
25	>16:37	15:42–16:37	<15:42
30	>16:54	15:59–16:54	<15:59
35	>17:11	16:16–17:11	<16:16
40	>17:28	16:33–17:28	<16:33
45	>17:45	16:50–17:45	<16:50
50	>18:02	17:07–18:02	<17:07
55	>18:19	17:24–18:19	<17:24
60	>18:36	17:41–18:36	<17:41

Your walking time .... min. : sec. ....

CALCULATION OF WALKING TIME FOR THE MEN'S WALKING TEST

Walking time in minutes : seconds for men

age	below average min. : sec.	average min. : sec.	above average min. : sec.
20	>15:07	14:08–15:07	<14:08
25	>15:24	14:25–15:24	<14:25
30	>15:40	14:41–15:40	<14:41
35	>15:57	14:58–15:57	<14:58
40	>16:13	15:14–16:13	<15:14
45	>16:30	15:31–16:30	<15:31
50	>16:47	15:48–16:47	<15:48
55	>17:03	16:05–17:03	<16:05
60	>17:19	16:21–17:19	<16:21

Your walking time .... min. : sec. ....

Test analysis: your fitness level

Which fitness type are you?

> Type A: Test time above average, test pulse low or in target range

You really are fit! Your capacity for endurance is excellent! The training plans for beginners and advanced would be under-challenging for you and would inhibit your motivation. Begin instead with a program for the super-advanced. Speed walking, Nordic walking or a light runner's training (see page 73) should challenge you to the proper extent.

> Type B: Test time average or above average, test pulse high

Your test pulse is higher than it should be. Although your fitness is up to par, you have to strain yourself to reach a good test result. Despite this, you can immediately start with the advanced training program on page 50.

> Type C: Test time below average or average, test pulse low

Your endurance level is sufficient. Did you not sufficiently exert yourself? Perhaps you also started too slowly. Repeat the walking test once again tomorrow and attempt to go faster. As an initiation into power walking the advanced program on page 50 can be recommended.

> Type D: Test time average or below average, test pulse substandard

Take advantage of the opportunity to become fit again! Speed walking is ideal for you and is the best option for doing something good for yourself, your conditioning, and your health. Begin with the walking program for beginners on page 49.

> Type E: Test time below average, test pulse high

You should do something for your health and fitness! Speed walking is the ideal program for this, as the load can be easily controlled even by complete beginners. However, speak to a doctor to make sure there are no health risks before beginning the training.

INFO

TARGET PULSE FOR WOMEN AND MEN IN THE WALKING TEST*

Age	Target pulse
20	160–190
25	156–185
30	152–181
35	148–176
40	144–171
45	140–166
50	136–162
55	132–157
60	128–152

Your test pulse .... Beats/min.

* The pulse during testing is higher than during training.

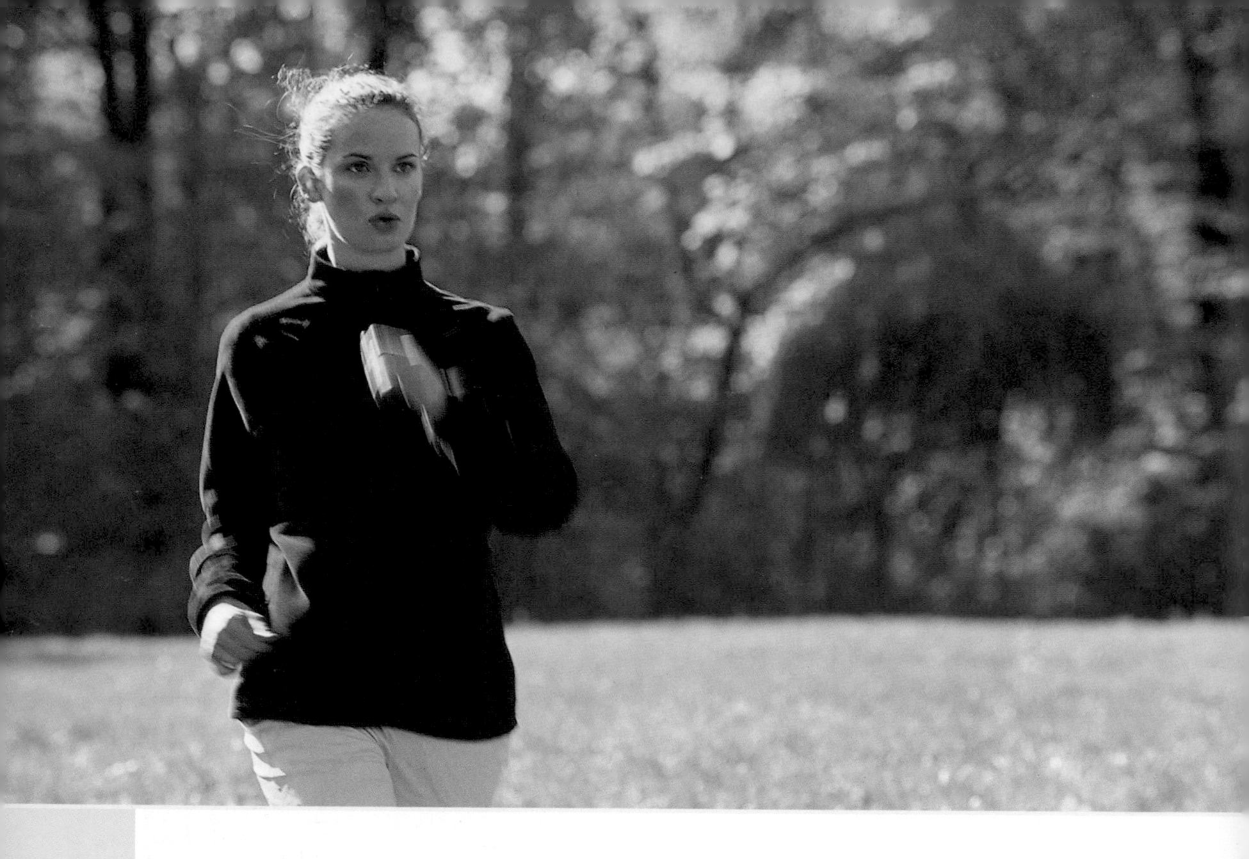

The proper walking technique

For correct walking, it isn't enough to just step on it. Only the proper technique turns strolling into the endurance sport called speed walking. You have to walk correctly if you want to increase your physical performance. You're playing it safe by training not just your legs but your whole body. But don't worry, that really isn't hard! You also become faster with the proper technique because you can put the strength of your legs to work in an efficient and energy-saving way. And another important plus: a correct walking technique is the best protection against overload and orthopedic complaints, such as those in the knee or spine. This is important most of all for people at risk, such as those who are overweight.

Legwork

With each step you place your foot heel first in front of you, then unfurl it over the entire sole to your toes. Then firmly push yourself up from the ground with your toes and set the heel of your other foot on the ground again. This motion is more easily accomplished if you imagine yourself actively pushing the ground under your foot away with each step.
While walking, the tips of your toes must point in the direction of travel. A slight turn of the feet in or out while doing this is completely normal.
As soon as you've gotten used to unfurling your feet, make sure that your knees are not completely locked when placing your heels down. Instead, always roll your foot with a slightly bent knee.

Pace length and frequency

The length of your steps during walking depends significantly on the speed and frequency of your steps. The faster you walk, the higher your pace frequency, and thus the number of steps, and the smaller your pace length. If, on the other hand, you take larger steps to walk a certain distance in less time, then the pace frequency automatically declines.

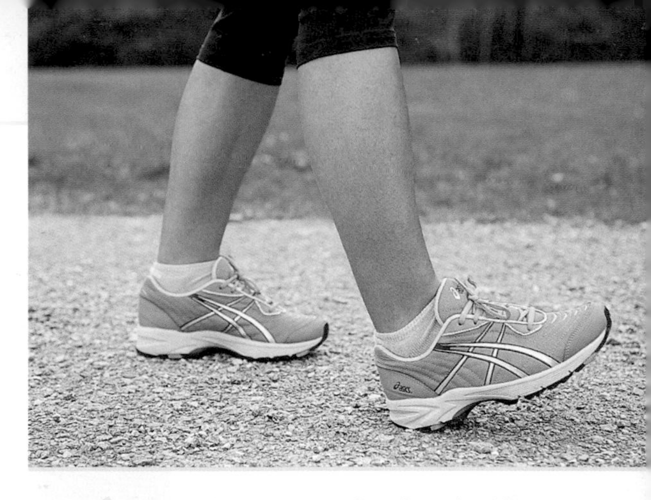

Always set your foot down heel first and unfurl it up to your toes.

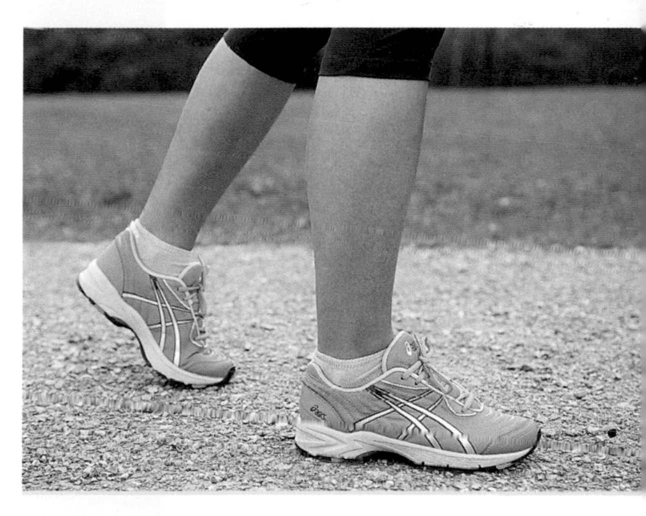

At the end of the unfurling motion press your body up from the ground with your toes.

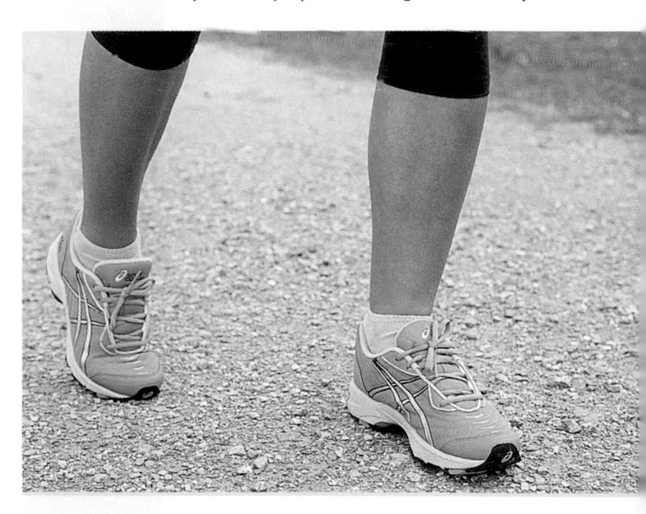

Your legs are parallel, the steps not too long.

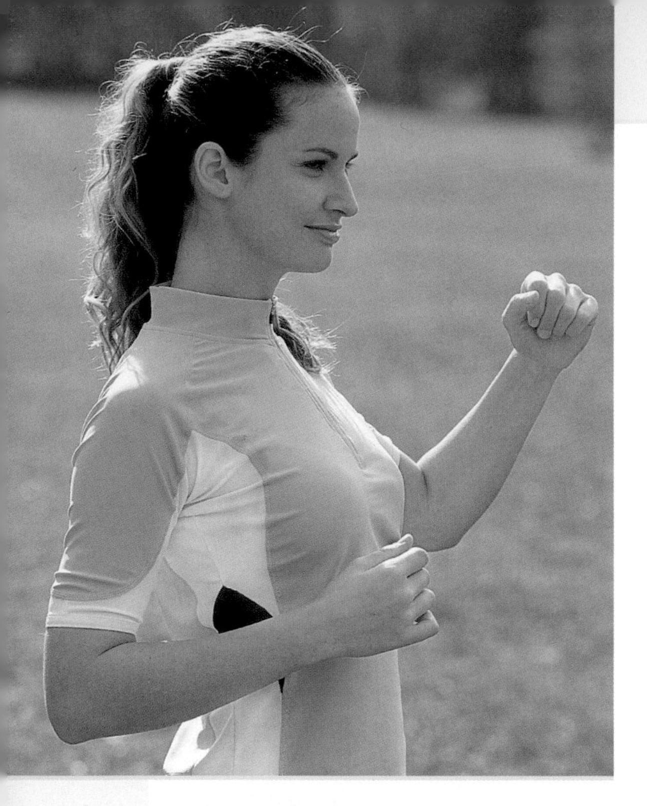

The arms form a right angle, hands are loosely closed.

Body posture

Once the foot technique has become second nature to you, you can pay more attention to correct body posture.
The upper body should be completely upright while walking. Pull your shoulders back and down so that your ribcage expands. For one, this ensures that you have room for the necessary breaths. It also prevents shoulder, neck, and back muscles from tensing up. Focus your eyes on the ground five to 15 feet ahead of you. This way you prevent tension in your throat and neck muscles as well, besides being able to dodge any obstacles in good time.

Active arms

Now actively integrate your arms into the cycle of movement. Stretched-out arms slow down the overall motion. Angle your arms at roughly 90 degrees and close your hands into loose fists. Keep your arms close to your body but move them rhythmically in a broad motion from your hips up to shoulder height. While doing this, arm motion should concentrate on the elbow's active backswing. Your arm will automatically swing forward again through the tension this creates in shoulder and chest muscles.
The arms swing back and forth in the direction of movement, but not at a slant. This would impair upright body posture and slow your pace. Swing your arms in direct opposition to your legs: put the left arm forward when you step forward with your right leg, and put your right arm forward when you step forward with your left leg. Make sure that your hands stay loose. Clenched fists indicate cramping.

Walking terrain

The consistency of your walking speed depends on the quality of the ground on which you're walking. Loose sand and rough gravel paths are not good. On the contrary, soft, springy forest paths, lawns, or non-asphalt park walkways are ideal.
If you live in the city it can hardly be avoided that you will have to walk part of the way on asphalt. For this reason as well, you should make especially sure that you have good shoes (see page 57) to protect your joints from unnecessary burden. During a seaside holiday take advantage of the opportunity to walk barefoot in firm sand. This way you will also get a beneficial foot massage for free.

Breathing

Your body must absorb more oxygen during times of exertion than during periods of rest. For this reason you should breathe deeper and faster while speed walking. Beginners especially run out of breath during walking. Just like speed walking itself, the correct breathing technique is a matter of practice.
You can actively support the respiratory process by breathing deeply and evenly in the rhythm of your walking pace, for example inhaling with three steps and exhaling again with the next three steps. Breathe in through your nose and out again through your mouth. This way your breath is warmed, humidified, and cleaned through your respiratory passages on its way to your lungs.

CHECKLIST

THE PROPER WALKING TECHNIQUE

1. Begin at a moderate pace.
2. Always place your heels on the ground with your knees slightly bent.
3. Roll your feet over the whole sole.
4. Set the points of your feet in the direction you're walking.
5. Angle your arms at 90 degrees and let them actively swing along from your sides.
6. Move your arms in direct opposition to your legs (right leg forward, left arm forward and vice versa).
7. Let your shoulders hang loosely.
8. Push your chest out while breathing.
9. Breathe consciously and evenly in and out.
10. Look ahead four to fifteen feet to be able to dodge any obstacles.

If you still run out of breath and have to try to compensate by breathing through your mouth, slowly reduce your tempo until you at last remain standing still. In most cases the reason for breathlessness is simply walking too quickly. Take a short break, during which you should try breathing not just through your mouth but through your nose as well. Sense how your breath slowly flows through your body to finally fill your lungs. When you have once again found your breathing rhythm, you can continue training.

Tempo and pulse

Depending on age, gender, and fitness level a person's pulse during times of rest runs 60 to 80 beats per minute. That means that our heart pumps one to two gallons of blood through the veins with every 60 to 80 beats. With exertion the pulse rises to what we call the maximum pulse (MP). Starting from the maximum pulse, there are various exertion levels for healthful training.
Thanks to a simple "pulse formula" you can determine your own optimal training pulse. The figures are valid for both men and women.

Pulse formula: Optimal training pulse

- Subtract your age in years from the number 220 (heartbeats). This will give you your maximum pulse (MP).
- Multiply this figure by 75 to 80 percent. This will give you your optimal training pulse frequency per minute (TPF) for circulatory training, at which you can always train on an aerobic level (right box).
- Multiply your maximum pulse by 60 to 70 percent. This will give you your optimum training pulse frequency per minute for the fatburning zone (slower pace).

Example: A 35-year-old woman has a maximum pulse of 185 (220 minus 35). Her optimal training pulse frequency for circulatory training thus lies between 139 and 145 (75 to 80 percent).
If she wants to lose weight she should train in the fat-burning zone (60 to 70 percent). Her pulse must then lie between 111 and 130. She should, however, speed walk for at least one hour. You've found your own proper walking when your training pulse lies evenly within the calculated figure according to this rule of thumb. In the course of regular training your fitness will improve and you will be able to walk faster and faster.

Instructions for measuring pulse

To manually measure your pulse you will need a watch with a second hand. This is how it works:

- Take a short break from your training and remain standing.
- Measure your pulse on your lower arm at the wrist. Practice applying a light pressure with your index, middle, and ring fingers to the point between the tendons and the bone of your wrist.
- When you feel your pulse, look at the watch and count the number of pulses for 15 seconds. Multiply this number by four to get your pulse per minute at the given time.
- If your pulse is higher than the optimal training pulse (see page 28), then slow down your training tempo until your pulse declines. If your pulse is lower than optimal, you can try walking a little faster.

Tip: Definitely get into the habit of measuring your pulse before walking. The reason is that if you run out of breath and your pulse is too high, it isn't all that simple to find it on your wrist.

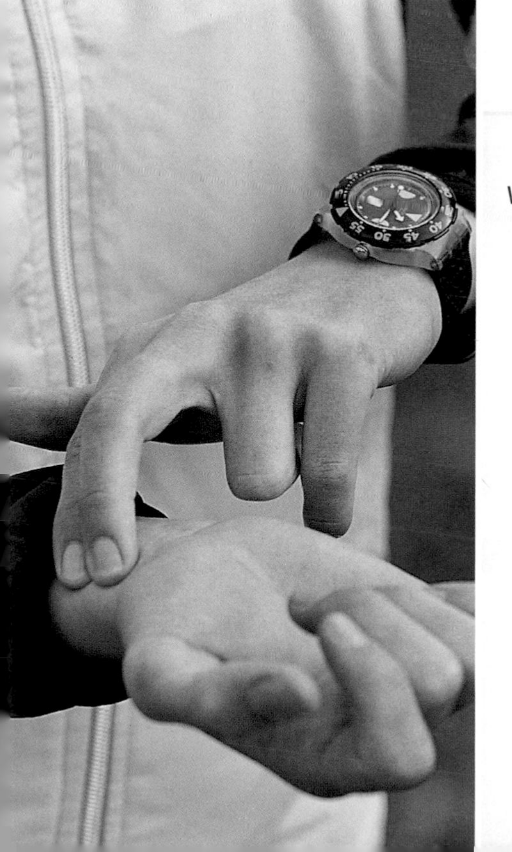

INFO

THIS IS HOW TO DETERMINE YOUR OPTIMAL WALKING PULSE

Age Woman Man	MP 220 minus age	Optimal TPF aerobic zone (75–80 %)	Optimal TPF fat-burning zone (60–70 %)
20	200	150–160	120 140
25	195	146–156	117–137
30	190	143–152	114–133
35	185	139–148	111–130
40	180	135–144	108–126
45	175	131–140	105–123
50	170	128–136	102–119
55	165	124–132	99–116
60	160	120–128	96–112

MP = Maximum Pulse, TPF = Training Pulse Frequency

Please note: Pulse figures can vary largely from person to person. If your pulse figures differ largely from the average figures, talk to a trainer or a doctor about this.

Pulse measuring device

If you want to make completely sure that your optimal training pulse remains constant during the complete program, train with the use of a pulse measuring device. It monitors your pulse with EKG precision without having to interrupt your training. Also, if for health reasons, for example after a heart attack, you are not allowed to exceed a certain pulse rate, a pulse measuring device is indispensable as an early warning system.

Aerobic and anaerobic training

Energy production in our muscular cells functions with oxygen (aerobic) or without (anaerobic) depending on how much we exert ourselves. If you train in the aerobic zone with moderate to medium intensity, your body takes the necessary energy mostly from fat deposits and not only from the speedily available carbohydrate reserves. Fat burning runs overtime then, because the mitochondria – the cellular power plants – have sufficient oxygen at their disposal.
If you are in good shape, this fat burning effect also functions if you have to exert yourself to a greater extent. Intensive exertion, however, such as a ten-second sprint to the bus, are only possible for most of us thanks to the energy gleaned from the anaerobic process. In this case no oxygen is necessary because your body is then making use of the carbohydrates stored in your muscle cells to achieve top speed. If, on the other hand, extreme exertion is sustained for a longer period, your muscles over-acidify due to a lactate surplus (i.e. too much lactic acid) from the breakdown of carbohydrates.
Your stamina will then subside and in most cases you will even be brought to a standstill.
Put in the context of speed walking, this means: the longer you want to walk, the lower your speed should be. Only then does aerobic energy supply function. You don't run out of breath, you do train your endurance, and metabolism of fats is particularly effective.

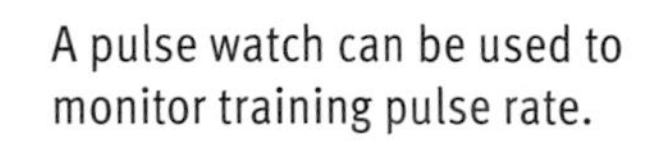

A pulse watch can be used to monitor training pulse rate.

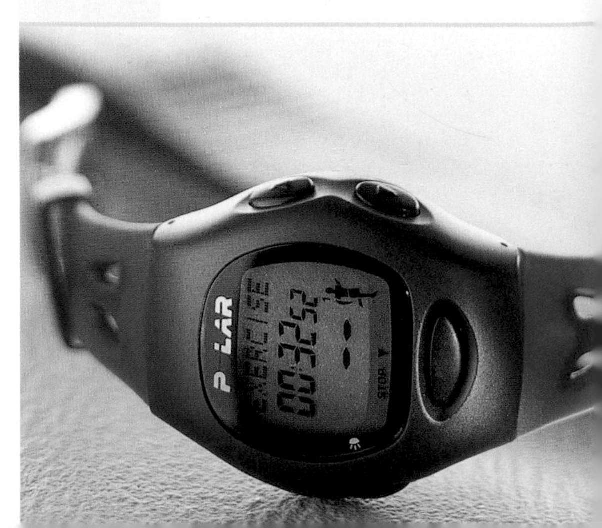

Warm up and cool down

Warming up and cooling down are essential components to every training. Pre-training exercises for mobility and loosening up prepare your body for the coming exertion. Stretching and relaxation exercises will help your training pass more smoothly.

Warming up

Stretching before training is not necessary because speed walking demands neither back-straining motions nor a large range of motion. After a short warm-up walk all that might be recommended is a short exercise in which you relax and rotate your shoulders and warm up your feet and ankles as well as your back for greater mobility.

Relaxing and Spinning Your Shoulders

Goal: Shakes off everyday stress and sets the tone for walking outside; aids against cramps and prepares you for active arm movement.

- Stand with slightly open legs.
- To relax your shoulders, rotate first your right, then your left shoulder back and forth a few times. Remain standing upright while doing this.

Shoulder tension

Goal: Relaxes the shoulders.

- Pull both shoulders up to your ears and hold this position for three seconds. Inhale while doing this. 1
- Then let your shoulders suddenly drop again. Exhale audibly while doing this to heighten the relaxation effect.
- Take a short break and repeat the exercise at least two more times.

1 3 times | every 3 sec.

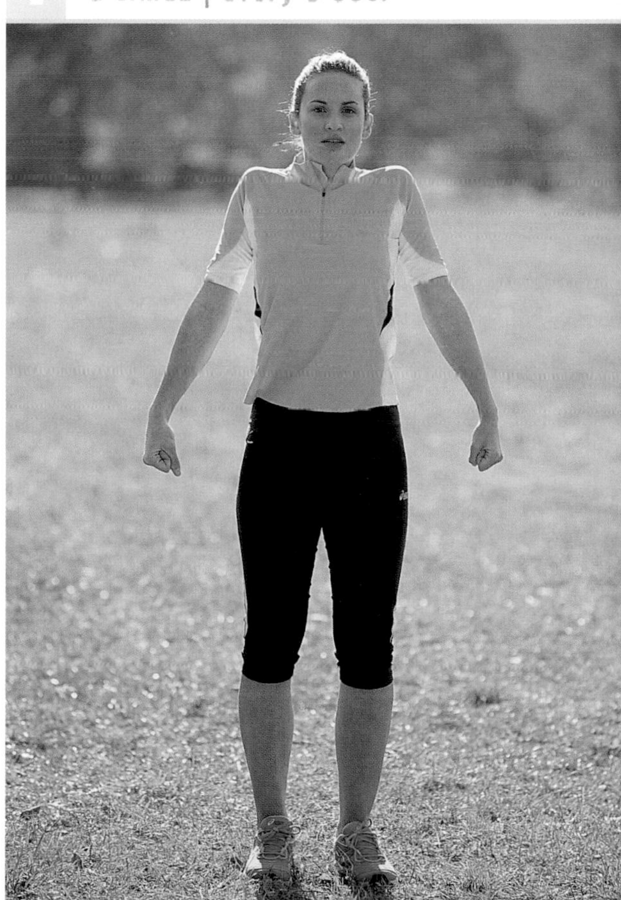

Ankle warm-ups

Goal: Helps cramping, warms up the joints, and prevents injuries.

- Slowly unfurl your feet, alternating from one to the other. Stand on the balls of your feet and back down again. Stand on your heels with your knees bent and back down again.
- Cross your feet, alternating between the right and the left. 2

Important: Bend your knees! In order to prepare for the proper foot movements necessary for speed walking, try to stand on your heels with your knees bent. The reason is that bent knees are essential for healthy speed walking without joint strain.

Mobilizing your back

Subsequently, the spine can be worked on. For this purpose, all exercises that aid cramps, supply vertebrae with nutrients, and introduce active relaxation are suitable . You should maintain each stretch for approximately 30 seconds.

Upper Back

- Stand upright, cross your arms over your chest and close each hand over the opposite upper arm.
- Raise your arms to shoulder height, take your head between

2 10 times

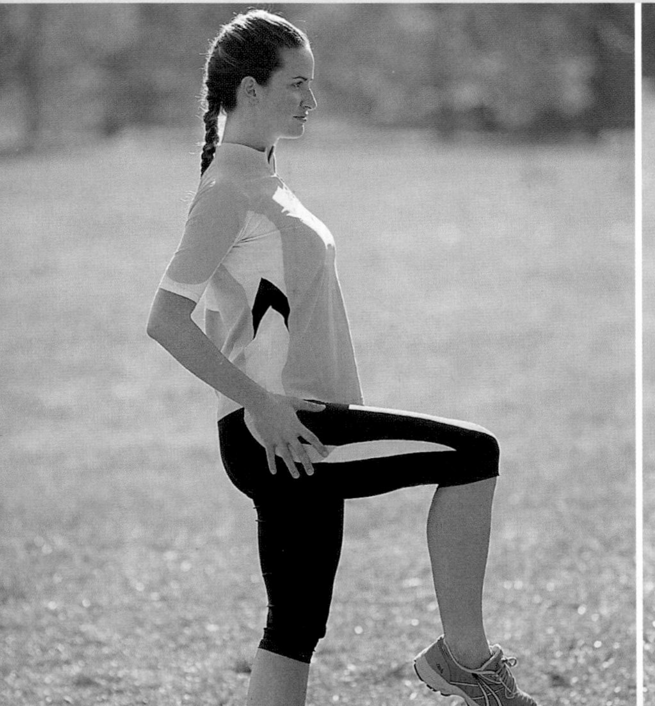

3 once | 30 sec.

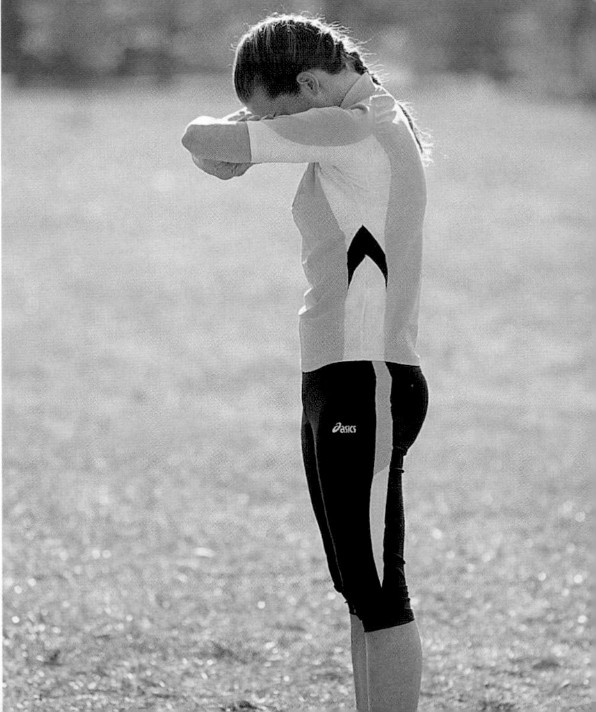

your arms and pull your arms and shoulders softly forward. Breathe easily in and out while doing this. 3

Shoulder blades

- Cross your arms in starting position and close each hand around the opposite shoulder blade. 4
- Now try to draw your shoulder blades inward as far as possible, so that your back is as rounded as possible. Do not forget to breathe while doing this.

Side tilting

- Stand upright once again and cross your feet so that the right foot is in front of the left one.
- Raise your arms over your head, lock your hands together, and turn your palms so that they point upward.
- Slowly tilt your upper body to the left, making sure not to hold your breath. 5
- Release the tension once again and turn back to the middle, continuing to breathe easily. Now set your left foot in front of the right one and stretch the other side.

4 once | 30 sec.

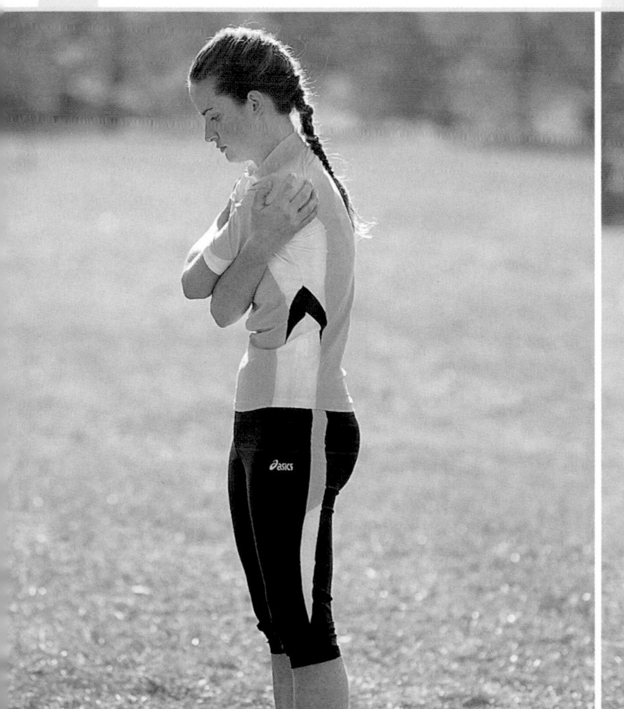

5 once | 30 sec.

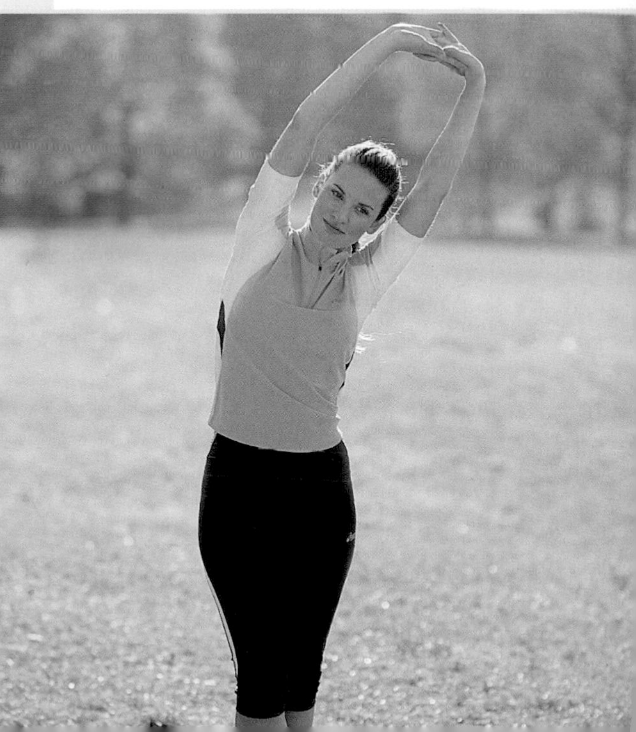

IMPORTANT!

THE PROPER WAY TO STRETCH

- Your stretching position is right if you can feel a slight pulling in your muscles.
- Maintain the stretch for about 15 seconds and then relax your muscles again.
- Repeat the alternation between stretching and relaxing a total of two to three times and then switch sides.
- Breathe easily and regularly during the whole exercise.

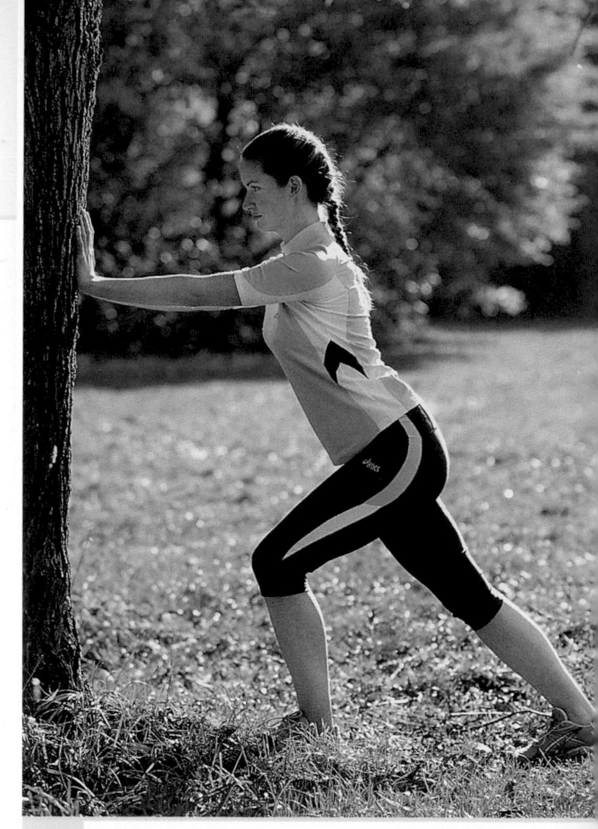

1 twice | every 15 sec.

Warm-ups and stretches

When you want to end your walking session, reduce your speed and continue walking for about 10 minutes at a slow pace before you come to a complete stop. Then end your training with a short stretching program. This way your muscles, which have been shortened by the strain on them, will be softly stretched back to their original length. Begin by stretching your calf muscles and the muscles in the front and back of your thighs. After this, stretch your chest, neck, hip, and lower back muscles.

Calves

- Take a small step forward and lean against the trunk of a tree with both arms. Your back leg should be extended, both heels touching the ground, your toes pointing forward.
- Swing your hips forward and try to push against the tree trunk with outstretched arms. The back leg should remain extended, without your heel rising from the ground. If you feel no tension, place your rear leg back further or extend the tips of your toes. 1
- Don't forget to switch sides!

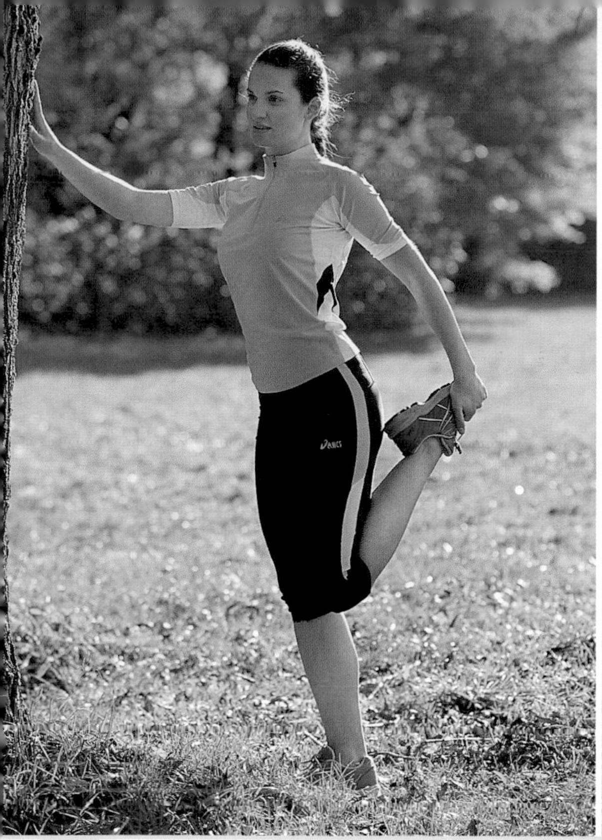

2 twice | every 15 sec.

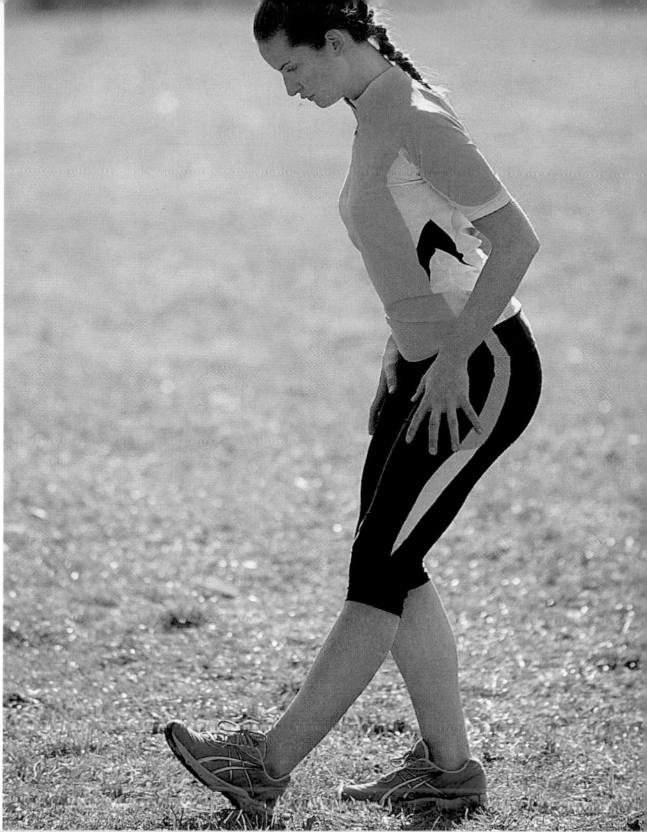

3 twice | every 15 sec.

Quadraceps

- Stand in front of a tree with slightly bent knees and lean onto it with your right arm. Remain standing upright while doing this. Tense the muscles in your stomach and rear to prevent saddle back.
- Angle your left leg backwards and hold on to the back of your foot with your left hand.
- Pull your foot back to your rear until you are able to feel the tension in the front of your upper thigh. Push your pelvis slightly forward. 2
- Don't forget to switch sides!

Hamstrings

- Take one step forward and raise your toes in such a way that only your heels are touching the ground. Carefully extend your knee. If it hurts to do this, you can bend your knee a little.
- Tip your pelvis back, push your butt back and out and bend your hip joint until you can feel the tension on the back of your upper thigh. Make sure that your back remains straight and you don't cause saddle back. 3
- Don't forget to switch sides!

Chest

- Stand an arm's length away from the side of a tree and grab onto the trunk with one hand sideways at shoulder height. The arm must be completely extended.
- Flex the muscles in your stomach and butt to avoid getting saddle back. Turn your upper body away from your arm until you can feel the tension in your arm and chest. 4
- Don't forget to switch sides!

Back of neck

- Stand upright with your legs slightly open and your knees a little bent.
- Your arms should hang loosely from your sides.
- Tilt your head forward and move both shoulder blades down at the same time. Feel the tension in your neck. 5

4 twice | every 15 sec.

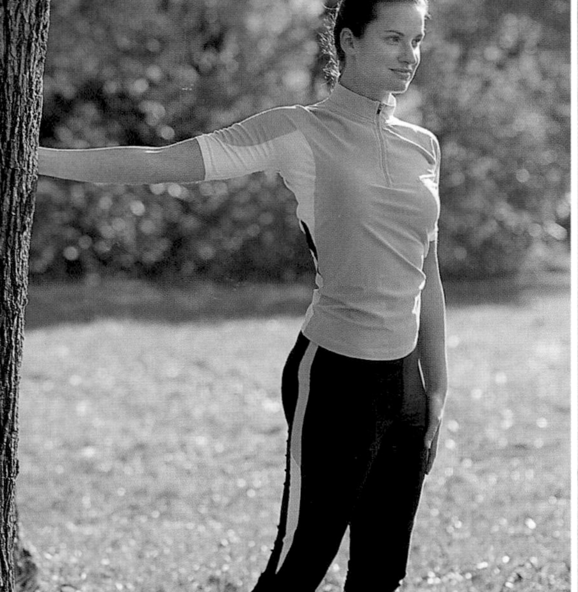

5 twice | every 15 sec.

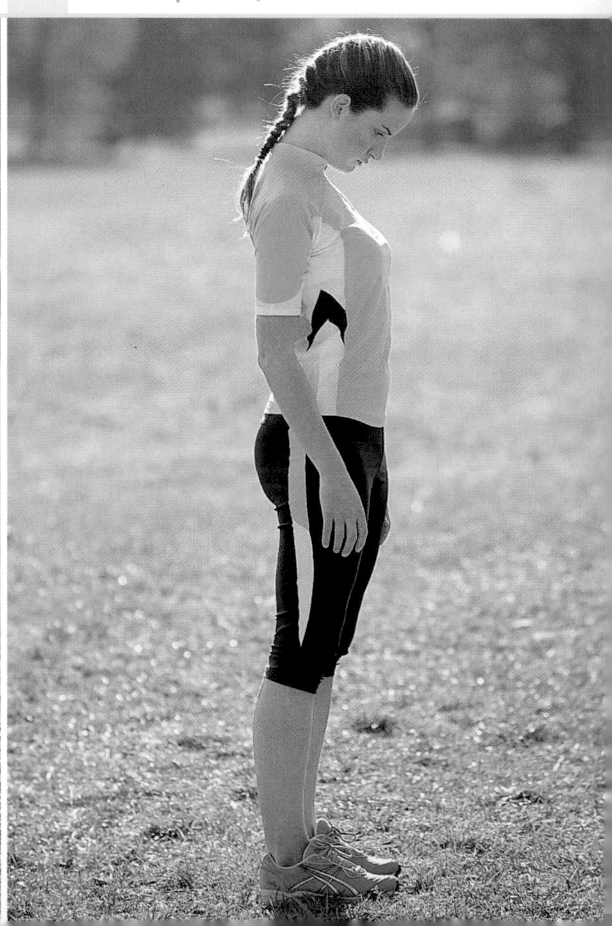

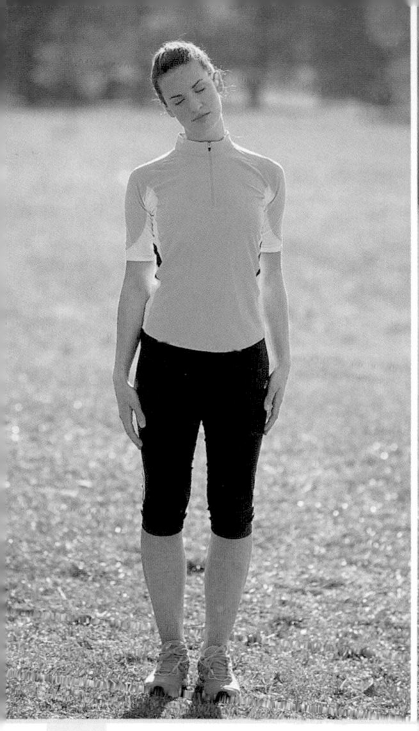

6 twice | every 15 sec.

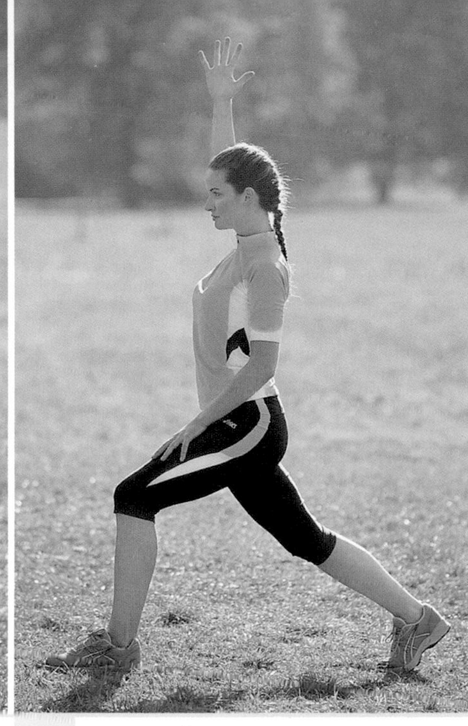

7 twice | every 15 sec.

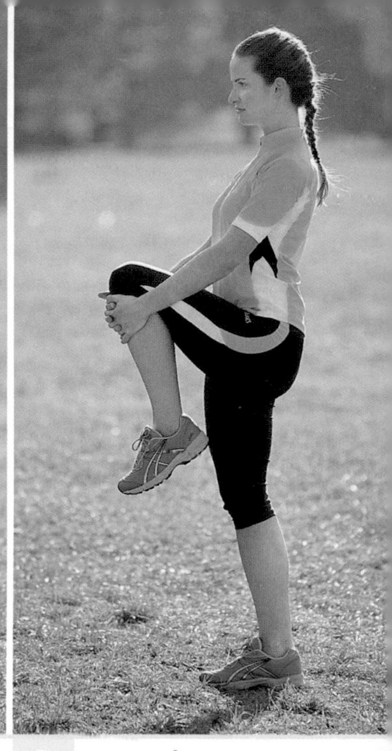

8 twice | every 15 sec.

Sides of neck

- Remain standing straight and tilt your head to one side. 6
- Push your other arm and shoulder down until you can clearly feel the tension in your throat.
- Don't forget to switch sides!

Hip muscles

- Take a big step forward with your left leg.
- Keeping your upper body straight, lean with your left hand on your left leg.
- Lift up your right arm with your fingers spread.
- Flex the muscles in your butt. Push your right hip down and stretch your right leg back far enough to feel it in your hips. 7
- Don't forget to switch sides!

Lower back

- Bend your leg and pull it up to waist height.
- Hold onto your knee with both hands.
- Push your knee forward into your hands until you can feel the tension in your lower back. Make sure that your back stays completely straight. 8
- Hold your head upright and look straight ahead.
- Don't forget to switch sides!

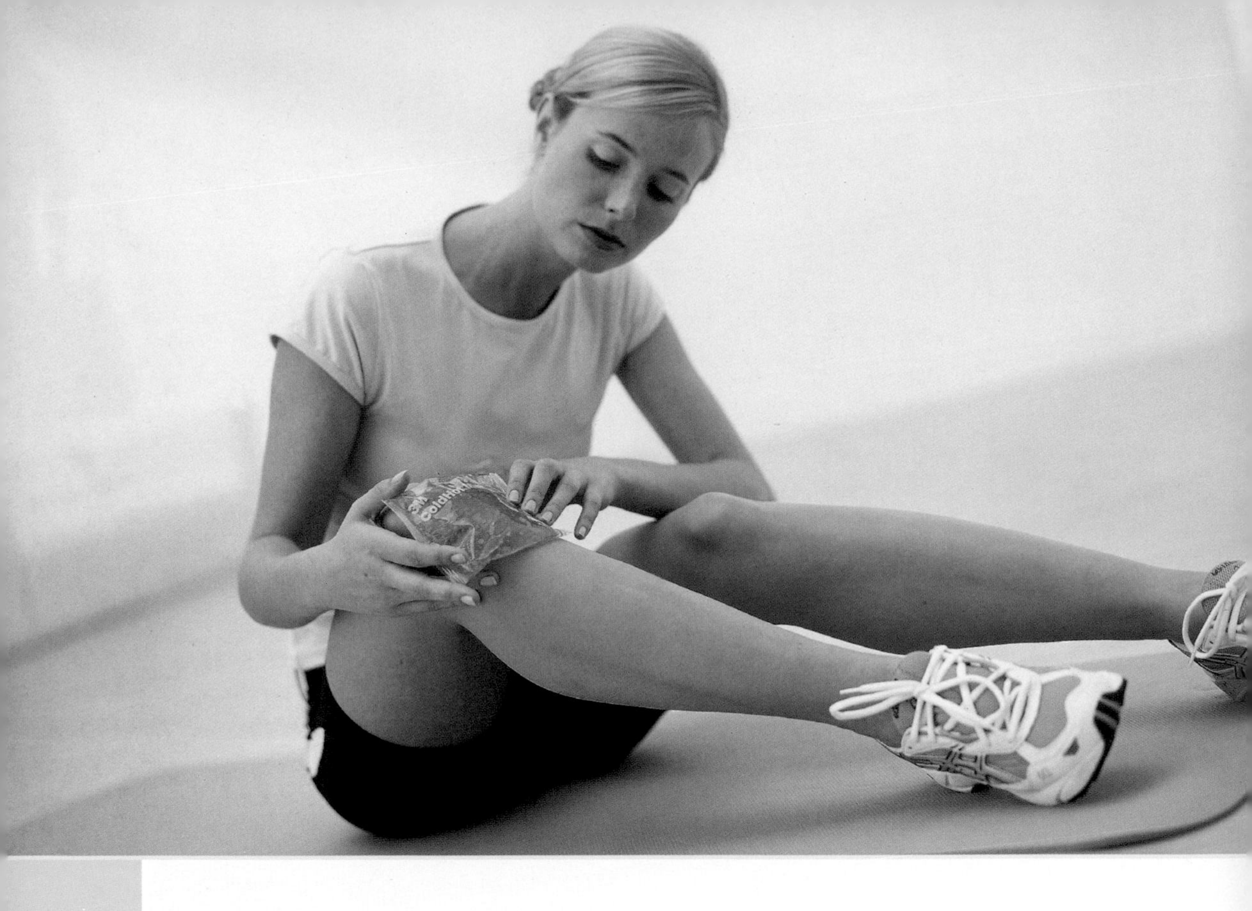

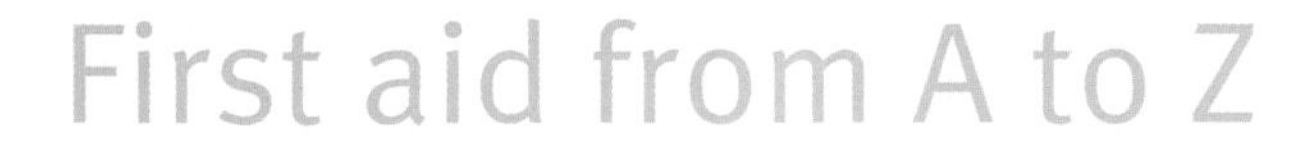

First aid from A to Z

Even though speed walking, compared to other types of sports, is very low-risk, under certain conditions typical sports injuries can arise. In addition, muscle cramps and joint pain might arise if you put too many demands on your body or if you increase the training load too quickly. Tiredness and lethargy are signs of over-exertion.

In most cases, you can contribute a lot yourself to prevention and treatment. Very important: Interrupt your training to avoid unnecessary movements or unnecessary strain. Set off for home and look for a doctor if the pain still hasn't subsided after the corres-ponding self-treatment.

Blisters

If your shoes or socks rub against your feet, painful blisters might arise. For this reason you should pay special attention to your shoes and wear special running socks.

To allow the fluid to escape from filled blisters, stick a sterilized needle into them. Put a special blister bandage (available from the pharmacy) over the wound. Such a bandage can also be used to guard high-risk spots on your feet from blisters.

A tip from the home pharmacy: Apply some therapeutic lavender oil onto the bandage before you place it over the blister. This will speed up the healing process.

Joint and muscle pain

Acute pain, for example in your knees or bones, can be cooled directly after training with a sack of ice or an ice pack around which you can wind a handkerchief.

Chronic pain, on the other hand, should be treated with heat, a warm shower for instance, infrared light, or an electric pillow. If the pains do not subside or if they continually return despite regimented training and other preventive measures, you should see a doctor.

Circulatory disturbances

Frequent causes of circulatory problems after walking include an overly high walking tempo and dehydration. For this reason you should monitor your training pulse and drink a pint of mineral water or sparkling fruit juice before you train.

While walking long distances under high temperatures it is recommended to continuously hydrate yourself. Per hour you should drink about a quart of not overly cold fluids in small swallows. You can carry a plastic bottle in a fanny pack or wear a small drink pack with a straw on your back.

TIP

SALTWATER COMPRESSES

If you frequently suffer from joint pain or contusions, it is recommended to always keep a saltwater compress near at hand. Dip a dish towel in strongly salted water, wring it out, and freeze it. The advantage: the salty ice melts more slowly and thus soothes longer.

How to recognize a circulatory disturbance

The first signs of a circulatory disturbance are the following:

- pale, cold, inflamed, or hot skin,
- a quick or racing pulse,
- nausea,
- dizziness, anxiety,
- loss of consciousness,
- cold sweat,
- freezing sensations.

By all means, pay attention to these signs because a disturbance of your vital functions as a result of oxygen depletion can have serious health consequences .

TIP

FIRST AID KIT FOR POWER WALKERS

If you want to play it safe you can put together a small first aid kit which can fit in a hip pack without any problem. This is what belongs in one:

- a cold pad, which cools when creased (available in pharmacies)
- sterile wound ointment
- a package of bandages
- gauze bandages
- adhesive bandages

This helps

If the first signs of a circulatory disturbance make themselves known, immediately reduce your speed and then come to a complete stop. If weather conditions permit, lay flat to the ground and put your legs up high. Open overly tight clothing and fan yourself if your skin feels hot. If possible, sprinkle yourself with water.
Try to keep yourself warm if you're shivering. However, you should not use external heat such as heating pads. Use clothing and blankets instead.

Muscle cramps

Many laypersons still believe that a muscle cramp is caused by a buildup of lactic acid in the muscle. This is actually not true. Muscle cramps arise because of very fine tears in muscle tissue. These small tears are painful but not, dangerous. If the injury has healed after two days, then the symptoms have disappeared as well.
You should not massage the painful parts. Only soft, stroking pressure and heat treatment (infrared light, warm baths, sauna) are permissible. Do not resume speed walking until the pain has subsided.

Because muscle cramps are always a result of too intense training, you can easily prevent them: adjust the walking load to fit your individual fitness level and only slowly increase the training intensity.

Shin pain

In the case of speed walking beginners, the muscles on the front of your shins have to get used to the unfamiliar strain. Ice or a cooling pack will help to soothe the pain. Cut back on your training in any case and walk at low speed so that your muscles can slowly grow. A false positioning of the ankle can also be a cause of shin pain. In this case you should check at an athletic store to see if you are wearing the proper shoes for speed walking. You can also stretch the muscles in your shin by placing the tips of your toes on the ground and carefully stretching your foot forward.

Side pains

In the case of overly heavy or irregular breathing, side pains may arise. Presumably, the cause is insufficient circulation in your mid section. When side pains arise, come slowly to a standstill and do an equalizing breath exercise from Qigong, such as the "Calming Down" exercise (page 107).
With complete exhalation old carbon dioxide is released from the body. In this way more oxygen can be brought in, bound to your blood, and carried to your muscles to compensate for the oxygen deficit.

Sprains, contusions, and strains

Sprains, contusions, and strains can be recognized by the following signs:

- pain,
- swelling,
- relieving postures,
- skin discoloration and
- limited movement.

If the pain does not subside, you should see a doctor to rule out a hemorrhage or torn ligament.

First aid

In any case you should rest the leg in question and place a compress on it. Closed injuries can be cooled with ice or a cold pack. To avoid cold shock, place a piece of cloth beforehand on your skin or wrap the ice in a hand towel or wash-cloth. You can try an arnica compress as well: dip a cloth in a half pint of water in which a tablespoon of arnica essence has been mixed. Or rub arnica salve into the spot twice a day.

Sufficient hydration effectively prevents variety of complaints

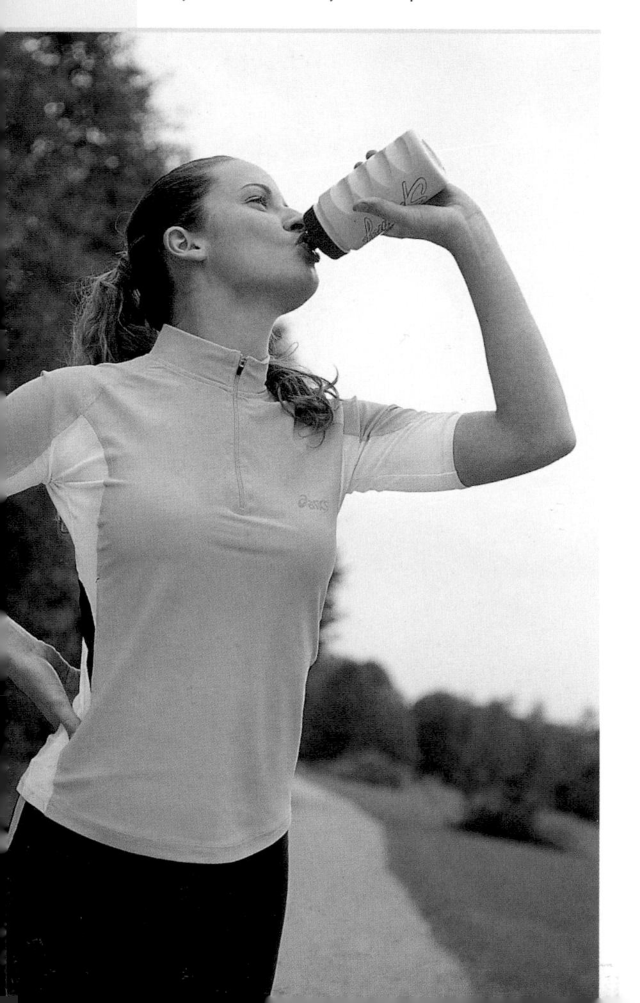

Calf cramps

Calf muscles can cramp up from one moment to the next through over-exertion or dehydration. First aid for this entails generous stretching (see page 34) and relaxing massages. If you have a tendency toward calf cramps, you should drink plenty of fluids and possibly take magnesium tablets as a preventive measure.

Wounds

Bleeding and wounds, for example after a fall, always accompany damages to skin as well as pain. Additionally, dirt or foreign particles, such as small stones, wood, or glass splinters might be in the wound, which pose a danger of infection.

What should you do?

When blood is flowing, many people get woozy in the stomach.
To prevent a shock, sit or lie down and breathe deeply and easily from your belly. Keep the injured body part high to slow the bleeding. If the wound begins to bleed again at home, or is still bleeding, place a sterile bandage on it and staunch the bleeding with a tourniquette. In the case of continued bleeding and foreign

particles in the wound you must go to the doctor. Under certain conditions, you should also get a fresh tetanus shot.

Leg aches

If your legs are sore after speed walking, the cause might possibly be overly intensive training or perhaps dehydration. For this reason you shouldn't increase your training load too quickly and should drink enough before, during, and after walking, especially mineral water or fruit juice spritzers.
Either way, you should never forget to sufficiently stretch after speed walking. This also works preventively against unpleasant leg complaints. The best exercises for this can be found on page 34.

Prevention!

The best first aid is the one that you don't even need. For this reason try to prevent possible difficulties during walking as much as possible:

- Walk on sufficiently broad paths with little unevenness. Avoid narrow forest paths with many roots (stumbling traps).
- The walking path should be well-lit, especially in winter.
- Pay attention to proper shoes and functional equipment (see page 56).
- Go without training in the case of extreme weather conditions such as heat, ice, or heavy rain. On days like this you might train on the treadmill of a fitness studio, for instance.
- Learn the Risk Check by heart on page 17.
- Monitor your heart rate while walking (page 62) and adapt your speed to your fitness level. Do not overdo it in your training sessions. It's best to walk neither to often nor too quickly, and reward your body with sufficiently long rests.

You can prevent against calf cramps with magnesium tablets.

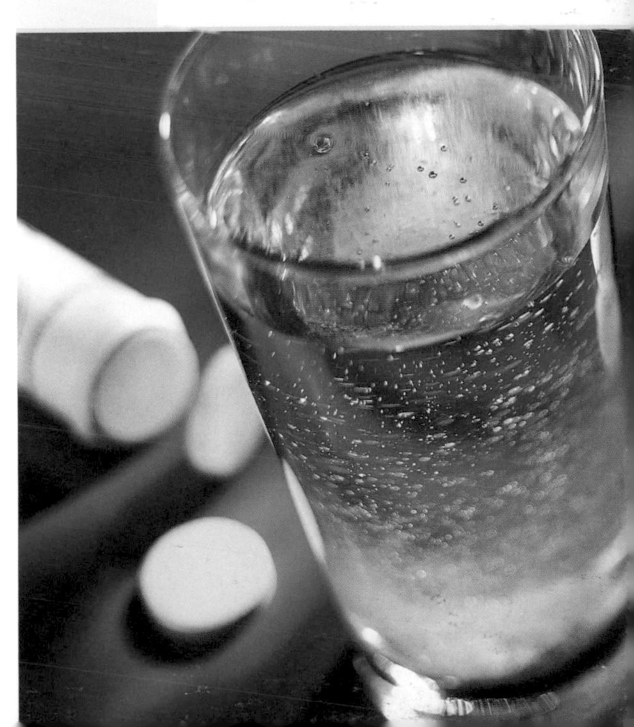

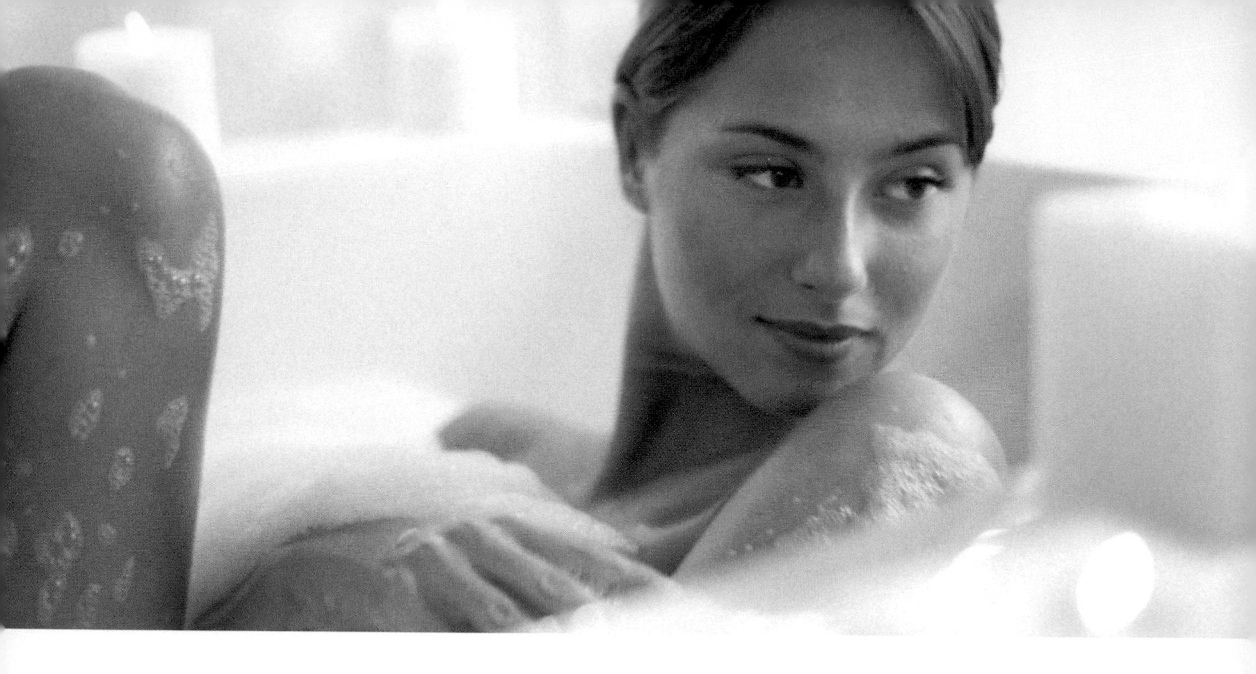

RELAXING CARE

Even if you don't overexert yourself and still walk only within your optimal heart rate parameters, you can break quite a sweat. For this reason you should relax and care for yourself after speed walking.

INVIGORATING SHOWER OR HEALTHY BATH

Always wait fifteen minutes before you shower or bathe. Your body continues to sweat during this time. Otherwise you might find that only a short while after showering you are soaking wet again.
Also pay attention to the proper water temperature – best about 96 °F. If the water is too hot, then your skin will dry out quickly. A shower gel with invigorating essential oils such as lemongrass, mint, or rosemary offers extra refreshment.
A true boon after heavy exertion: Just let the lukewarm water run down your spine for a few minutes. Or you can take a relaxing bath.

ALL-AROUND FRESH

A refreshing body powder will leave a pleasant sensation on your skin for the entire day after bathing or showering. Put some powder in a shaker or in a simple jar and use a powder puff to apply.

Peppermint body powder

Put one cup of rice starch in a jar. Dissolve 15 drops of peppermint oil in one teaspoon of vodka and drizzle this over the rice starch. Close the jar and shake it well to combine the ingredients. As the powder is drying, continue to occasionally shake the jar to prevent clumping. Sift it through a sieve into a tin.

FOR FEET AND LEGS

If your legs feel heavy after walking and your feet are hot, soothing lotions and foot baths will help.

Foot path for sweaty feet

Brew two teabags of sage tea in one cup of boiling water. Let the tea infuse for ten minutes before placing it in a bowl with a couple pints of lukewarm water. Let your feet soak in the mixture for ten minutes.

For heavy feet and legs

Combine two to three drops each of peppermint oil and menthol essence with a couple tablespoons of cold whole milk. Stir it all together and salve your feet with the mixture.

AROMA MASSAGE

Light massages and rubs with aroma oils help against tension and muscle cramps. The reason is that fragrant oils don't only stimulate the senses but have a physiological effect as well. To make your own massage oil you will need 1.5 ounces (100 ml) jojoba oil and pure aroma oils (available at pharmacies or from health food stores).

For painful muscles and ligaments

Add 20 drops each of aromatic eucalyptus, tea tree, and clove oil to to 1.5 ounces of jojoba oil.

For bruises

Combine 1.5 ounces of jojoba oil with 20 drops each of aromatic lavender oil and arnica oil.

Basic massage

- Always massage towards the heart – from bottom to top.
- Massage the legs with long strokes. Leave the area around the joints alone.
- Only massage forcefully enough that it stills feels pleasant.

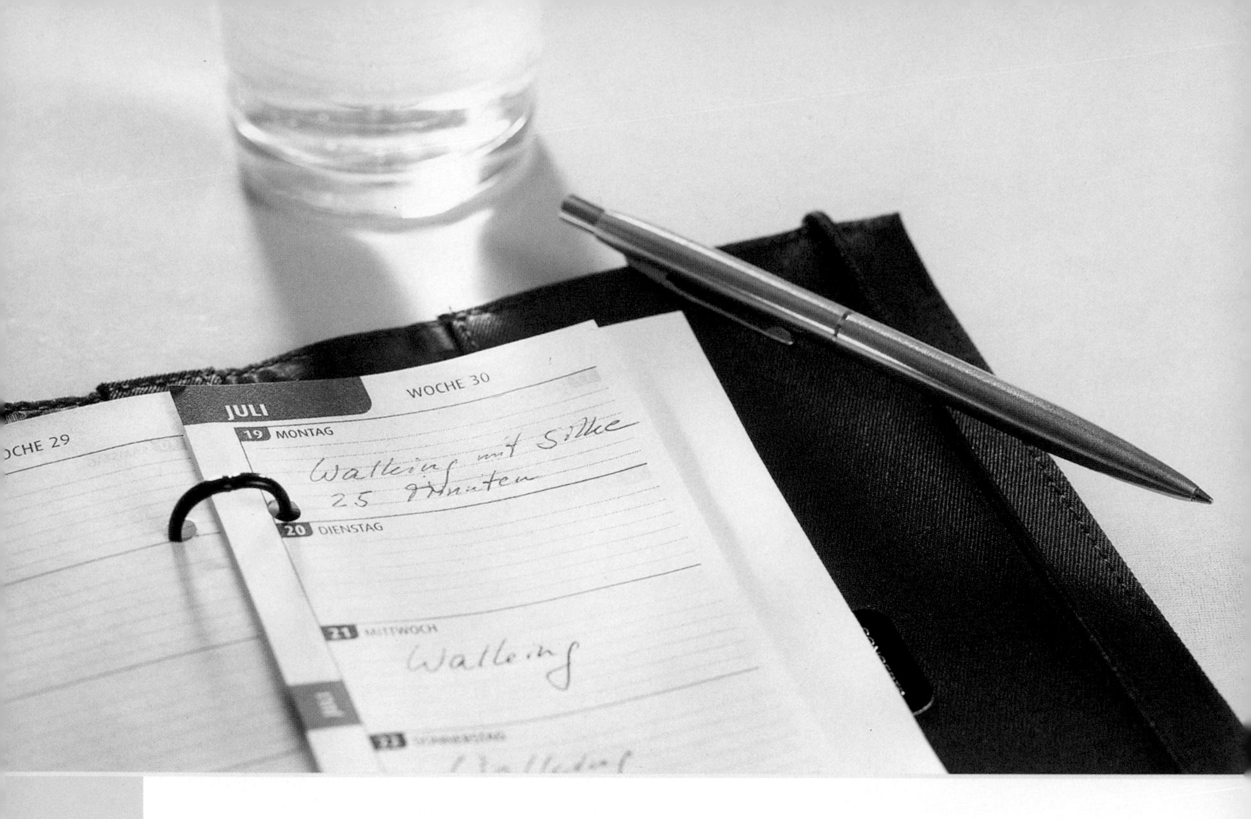

Speed walking training program

With speed walking, training length and frequency also play a decisive role. Only regular and sufficiently long power walking has a healthy effect. Our muscles unfortunately have no memory. If you want to condition yourself better or lose weight through speed walking, then you must train regularly. But caution: Even if your motivation is especially high in the first weeks, do not overdo it! Slowly adapt training length to your fitness level.

The reason for this is that a gradual increase to training enables you to maintain a stable physical capacity for longer than if you push it in a short time. Do not forget either that your body must be given sufficiently long periods of rest between training sessions. Only in this way is it able to recuperate and achieve the processes of adaptation that are so beneficial to your health.

Training plan

If it has been years since you've played a sport or have not been physically active in that time, just one power walking session a week can have a positive effect on your well-being. You should go speed walking two to three times a week, however, to optimally improve health and lose weight.
Of course, you can just go at it and follow your subjective intuition. But you can also follow a specific training plan to ensure that you are neither under- nor over-challenged. The first commandment in this case is: Take it easy! Walk during the first weeks for 30 minutes each week. Once your body has gotten somewhat used to the exertion you can increase the load – to three to four rounds each week, each of which should last about one hour. You can see on page 50 how your training plan can look.

Planning in your time-outs

After an hour of speed walking you will generally feel comfortably exhausted and your capacity is lower than before speed walking. Your body needs time to recover so that it can compensate for the tiredness and become physically capable once again. Speed walking has a healthy and invigorating effect only within a balance of exertion and relaxation. Your body makes additional energy reserves available in its regenerative phase so that during the following training session you will be capable of higher achievement. The result: your endurance increases.

Don't overdo it!

Beginners as well as starting again will be able to determine an improvement in their physical capacity after only a short time. But caution: The circulatory system and your nerves and muscles adapt much more quickly to the demands of power walking than do tendons, ligaments, bones, and cartilage. These require a longer constructive phase to be able to sustain the unfamiliar strain that speed walking provides.

TRAINING TEMPO AND LENGTH

Training intensity (speed) and length (distance covered) exist in inverse proportion to each other. The longer the training distance, that is, the lower your speed should be. Also, the shorter you walk, the faster.

IMPORTANT !

To ensure that the chance of injury remains low, the rule of thumb for speed walkers is: Begin moderately and do not put too much strain on your body at one time. Increase your walking load at a continual rate during the second phase. Do not reduce training if you have technically reached your goal for distance, speed, and frequency of training. Instead, try to maintain these figures over a longer period of time.

Pay attention to your limits

If you train with consideration of age and fitness level, and plan enough breaks into your training schedule, the threat of over-exertion during speed walking is almost nonexistent. If, however, your body is put under too much strain, it will send clear signals that you are well-advised to pay attention to. Especially important: Do not measure yourself against others or against unrealistic fitness goals but rather put together your own personal walking program. Listen to your inner voice when doing this. You know best what does your body good. Joint pain, a racing heart or muscle cramps, for instance, are certain indications of over-exertion. In these cases you should immediately reduce your speed and significantly decrease your training.

Pains

Pains that arise during or after training can be a sign of over-exertion. You should end your training session if your joints or muscles are hurting. Acute pains or strains are easily handled on your own (see page 38). If the pains don't recede after some time, however, you should go to a doctor.

Recessive joint pain

Joint pain that disappears during speed walking is a sign that you are not getting enough exercise in your day-to-day routine. Even if, as in this case, the exercise causing this pain might be seen as positive, you should still pay attention to it and in some circumstances consult a doctor about it.

Colds, etc.

You must absolutely refrain from speed walking if you have a cold, a fever, or acute inflammation. These infections usually run their course without any complications. They can, however, quickly expand to lung and cardiac inflammations under physical exertion.

Dullness and tiredness

If you feel worn-out and tired, this might indicate an excessive intensity in training. If you haven't given yourself a sufficient period of recuperation between two training sessions, this might lead to a decrease in capacity, expressing itself in dullness and lethargy. Interrupt your training to gather new strength!

Training plan for beginners

The walking program on page 50 was specially designed for the conditioning capacity of beginners and speed walking reinitiates.

It correlates with test result D in the endurance checkup on page 23. You will make quick progress if you stick to the program regarding the number of training sessions as well as session length and suggested pulse rate.
The pulse rates reflect your (yet) below-average capacity and the fact that you must first become acquainted with the increased exertion.

Weeks 1 to 4

To adapt your circulatory system to the increased load, walk during the first four weeks with a training pulse rate at 60 percent of your maximum pulse (see chart below).

INFO

TRAINING PULSE RATE FOR AGES 20–60

	Maximum Pulse	Training Pulse Rate		
Age	**100 %**	**80 %**	**75 %**	**60 %**
20	200	160	150	120
25	195	156	146	117
30	190	152	143	114
35	185	148	139	111
40	180	144	135	108
45	175	140	131	105
50	170	136	128	102
55	165	132	124	99
60	160	128	120	96

Two training sessions of 15 to 30 minutes each guarantee that you will not over-exert yourself, that your tendons and ligaments will not be over-strained, and that you won't lose your motivation to speed walk immediately after. Pay attention to the proper walking technique, especially in the beginning phase, to achieve the optimum training effects.

Weeks 5 to 8

In the following four weeks you should not strain your training pulse rate beyond 60 percent. The physical capacity you achieved in weeks 1 to 4 stabilizes during this time. You should increase, however, the number and length of training sessions: two to three walks per week of 30 to 45 minutes each should now be no problem for you.

Weeks 9 to 12

Beginning with the ninth week you should raise your pulse rate to 75 percent of your maximum pulse. At this level of exertion the optimal balance between oxygen intake and oxygen consumption is ensured – over-exertion is almost completely excluded. Walk for 45 to 60 minutes three to four times a week.

Week 13 and Beyond

After your 12-week training you should take the endurance checkup once again (page 20). You will definitely notice that your stamina has improved: you can walk faster and you feel less exhausted than at the start of training. This is the best motivation! If you want, you should be able to continue training with the program for advanced walkers.

Training plan for advanced walkers

If you have reached fitness level B or C in the exertion checkup (page 23), then you can begin right away with

INFO

TRAINING PLAN FOR BEGINNERS AND REINITIATES

Weeks	1–4	5–8	9–12
Optimal Heart Rate (% of max. pulse)	60 %	60 %	60–75 %
Training Time per Session (in minutes)	15–30	30–45	45–60
Sessions per Week	2	2–3	3–4

the program for advanced walkers. But caution: Even if you are highly motivated, you should stick to the given figures regarding training length, sessions, and pulse rate.

Weeks 1 to 4

You already have enough endurance to walk two to three times a week from the start. Begin at a moderate pace with a training pulse rate of 60 percent of your maximum pulse rate. By the end of the third week at the latest you should have reached a pulse rate of 75 percent. If you walk for 20 minutes at the start of training, this is perfectly sufficient. Afterwards, increase this time to 45 minutes over the course of your training.

Weeks 5 to 8

In this phase you will increase the length and frequency of your training. Walk three to four times a week for 30 to 45 minutes each session. Your heart rate should remain unchanged, ideally at 75 percent.

Weeks 9 to 12

In the 9th to 12th weeks you will again train at a pulse rate of 75 percent. Then increase your training time once again. Bring it up to 45 to 60 minutes per training session, and then raise your training frequency by 3 to 5 times.

Week 13 and Beyond

Test your endurance again after 12 weeks (page 20). You will probably find yourself already under type A in the evaluation. Of course, this does not mean that you can't continue speed walking as before. You can also try other walking variants such as Nordic walking or light running (page 73).

INFO

TRAINING PLAN FOR ADVANCED WALKERS

Weeks	1–4	5–8	9–12
Optimal Heart Rate (% of max. pulse rate)	60–75 %	75 %	75 %
Training time per session (in minutes)	20–45	30–45	45–60
Sessions per week	2–3	3–4	3–5

THE BEST MOTIVATIONAL AIDS

"I speed walk because it's fun and because I feel great afterwards!" This attitude is the best prerequisite for your body to get walking with the highest possible stamina. No one is always that motivated, however. Off-time – who isn't familiar with it? Sometimes you can use the following motivational aids.

OWL OR NIGHTINGALE?

Not a morning person? Of course, if you have a hard time getting out from under the sheets in the morning, speed walking before starting work takes a lot of self-motivation. In this case, you should walk after work. And the reverse holds true: If your energy disappears drastically in the evening, do your training session in the morning instead. Try in any case to always train at the same time of day. This way your body can adapt itself and have its energy reserves ready.

CREATE RITUALS

Create your own rituals and include speed walking as an essential component of these. Make your rounds in the morning, for instance, before breakfast and stop by the baker's afterwards to get your fresh rolls. Or you might draw a relaxing bath for yourself after training in the evening, to get rid of the last remains of daily stress.

FIND NEW PATHS

Day in, day out the same path and same faces? Nothing brings a change of pace to speed walking faster than a new route! Especially on weekends you can pick out a particular path to travel.

SEEK OUT LIKE-MINDED COMPANIONS!

At a moderate speed walking pace you can carry on a conversation without a problem – the time will fly by. Also, the "inner couch potato" can often be more easily overcome if you're afraid of leaving your training partner in the lurch. You can also join an organized speed walking group, such as from the local community college.

MUSIC DOES IT!

Music helps to switch off your everyday cares, and gives you plenty of new pizzazz. So put those headphones on, put in your favorite music, and off you go! There is also special walking and jogging music available that is set in three-quarters time. This can help you to better maintain a breathing and walking rhythm – breathing in with three steps, out with three steps.

WALKING WITH YOUR FOUR-LEGGED FRIEND

A dog is the best motivational aid for speed walking. A dog always wants out, and must get out as well, regardless of whether the sun is shining, it's raining, or its storming. If you don't have your own dog, you most likely know people who would be happy to not have to take their animal out on walks themselves.

SPEED WALKING DIARY

Write down your experiences with speed walking as well as your personal data – not every time, but now and again. If you have some spare time, just leaf through your walking diary a little. What have you achieved in the past weeks and months? How have your walking time, stationary, and walking pulse rates changed? Have you lost weight? Once you see all those small successes, you will definitely find it easier to convince yourself to continue your walking.

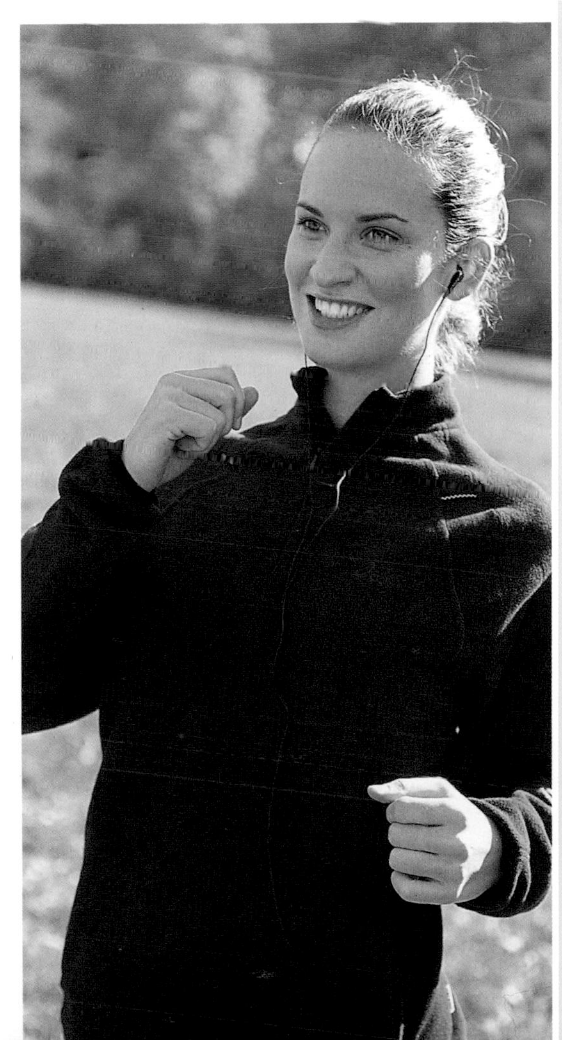

DATE YOURSELF!

Don't look at speed walking as a bothersome chore, but rather as a date with yourself, an hour in which you do something really good for yourself. Plan this "date" into your day just as you would plan a meeting with your friends. Put a thick X in your calendar and stick to this date.

Indoor training on a treadmill

Training on a treadmill at the fitness studio is a good alternative if the weather is bad, if you don't enjoy training alone, or if you are hesitant about walking after dark. The biggest difference: instead of moving from one spot to the next, you're walking on top of a moving surface. In this case your walking pace depends on the speed you program into the treadmill display at the start of training. Of course, you can always change this speed according to whether your training pulse is too high or too low – all you have to do is push a button.

Posture and motion

The criteria for training on a treadmill are the same as those for walking in the outdoors. You only have to determine how high your speed must be so that you are training at your optimal heart rate. Move your arms exactly as you would when training outdoors. With your breathing there is no difference

You can walk "dry" in any weather on the treadmill of a fitness studio.

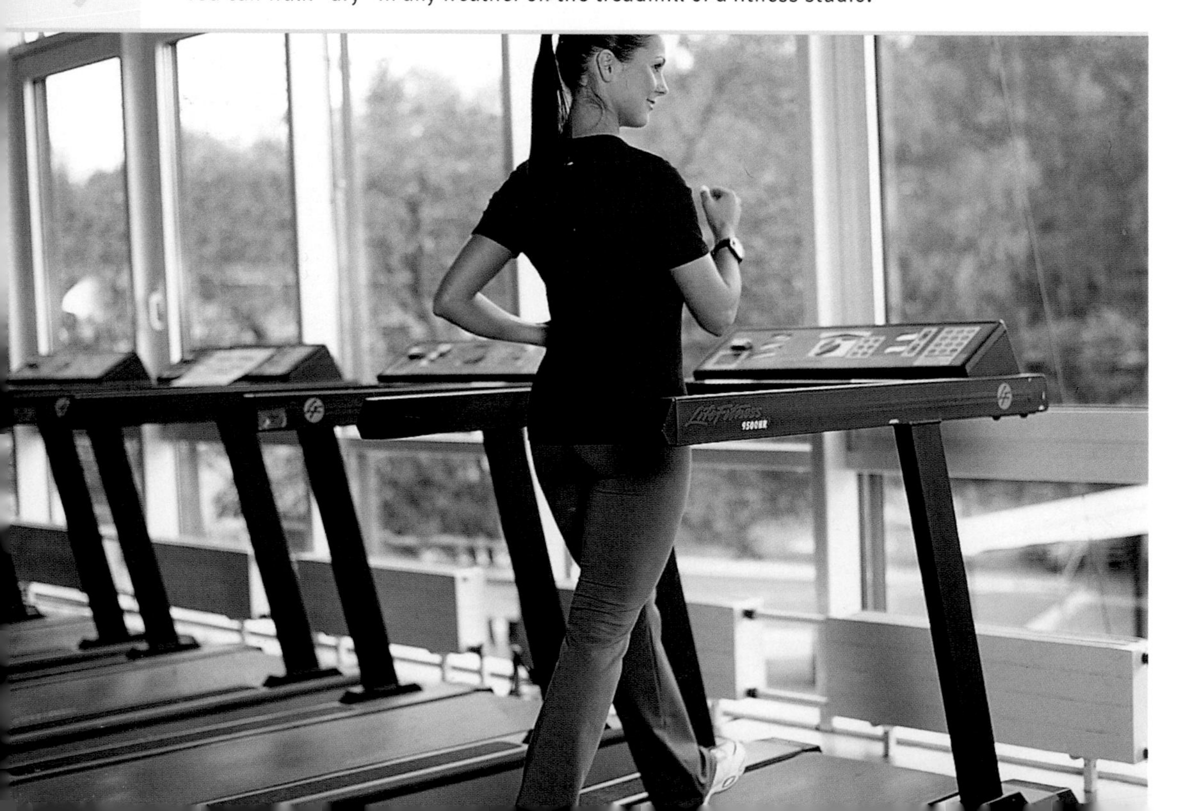

either. You should dispense with the practice of forcefully pushing off with your toes, however, because of the unstable surface. Walk in a loose and relaxed manner so that you don't get out of rhythm. And make sure you have especially good shoes to cushion the hard surface of the treadmill.

Technical equipment

You don't need a pulse watch to train on a treadmill. A built-in heart monitor displays the signals sent by the chest brace directly on a large monitor. The monitor should also show training time and speed as well as the fictional route's gradient and your calorie consumption.

Training advantages

Because a trainer is on site at the better fitness studios to consult you, power walking on a treadmill is ideal for anyone who has to train at a precise heart rate. A treadmill is also ideal for speed walking or competitive sports training because time, distance, and speed can be precisely adjusted. Training on a treadmill also allows you to easily have a conversation with your training partner or the person next to you. In many studios music and screens provide additional entertainment.

Walking test on the treadmill

If you have never walked on a treadmill before, take the time to get used to many of its particularities. As soon as you are fit enough to walk for 15 to 20 minutes at a speed of 3.5 to 5 miles per hour, you can take the 1.5-mile walking test. Program the treadmill and walk the distance as quickly as you can. While doing this make sure to measure your time and heart rate. Evaluate your results as you did in the endurance checkup on page 20. If you fall under type A, you can make your training more demanding by varying the gradient of the treadmill and walking uphill. If you fall under type E, get the advice of a fitness trainer so that he can develop a speed walking program for beginners on the treadmill for you.

CAUTION: DANGEROUS OBSTACLES!

A treadmill's moving surface also harbors a threat of injury for inexperienced treadmill walkers. The proper speed setting and heightened concentration while speed walking are the best preventative measures against stumbling, missteps, and spills.

IMPORTANT !

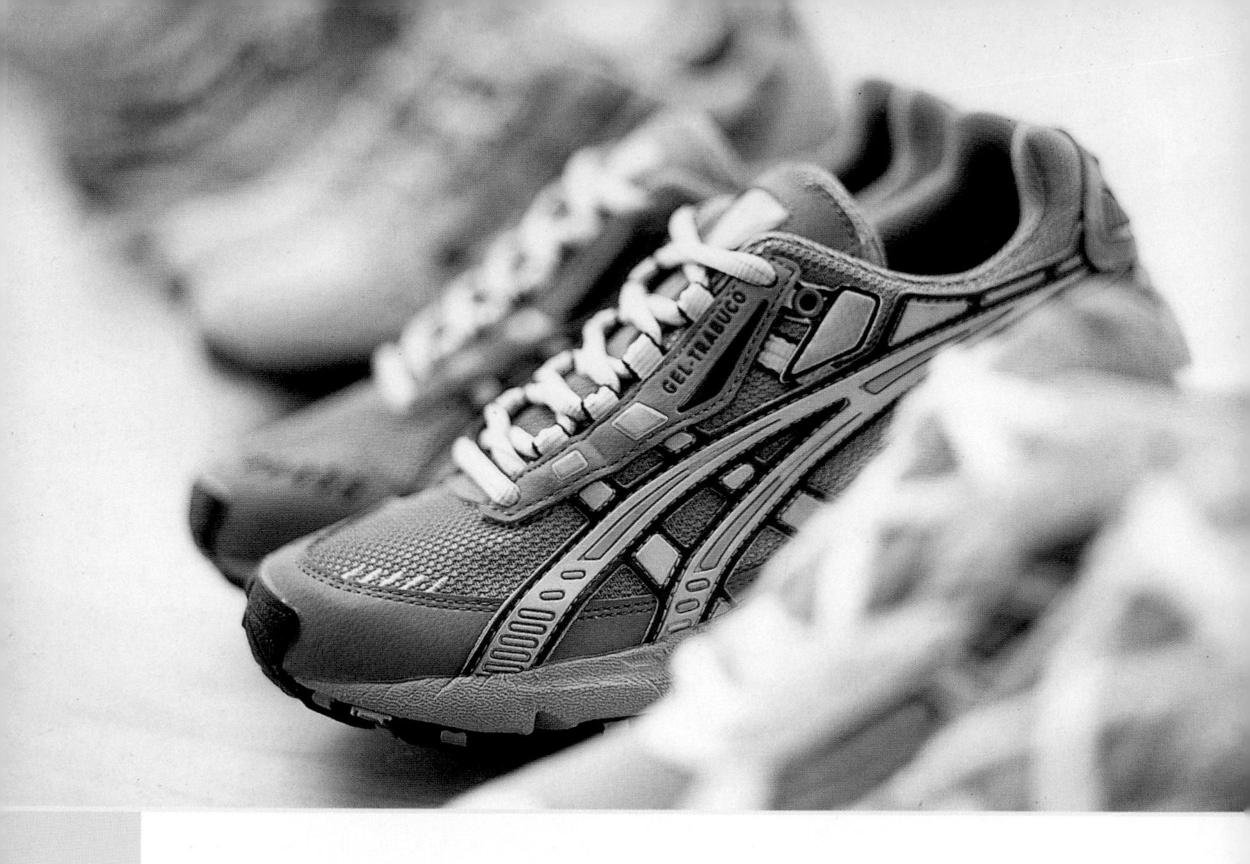

Shopping aid: Walking gear

Good shoes are the most important thing for speed walking. Speed walking is otherwise a sport for which no complicated gear is necessary. With the proper shoes and functional clothing you can actually start speed walking right away. But there is special clothing and a few accessories that make training more pleasant. In any case, you should make no compromises when it comes to your shoes. They are the foundation for all good walking equipment. They help to prevent possible damage to joints or ligaments. A good speed walking shoe is developed by the producer after an exact analysis of the cycles of motion and patterns of movement of the lower thigh, ankle joint, and foot to offer stability and optimal cushioning.

Shoes made to order

Despite their complicated construction, modern speed walking and jogging shoes are light. They guarantee the most natural freedom of motion for the foot with its 26 bones and 40 joints.
A good shoe must not inhibit movement but rather work with the foot in each phase of movement.
A shoe must sufficiently cushion the right spots and guide and stabilize the foot. Only in this way can it help to achieve complete potential and reduce risk of injury. Due to its slightly slanted shape, an asymmetrical sole, for instance, ensures a cushioned rolling motion from first contact with the ground. Peripheral indentations around the foot area divide the sole into several zones and guide the foot into its most natural movement. Innovative, precisely positioned gel cushioning systems under the heel and ball of your foot soften and disperse the forces that strain your joints when pushing off from the ground. While standing, the inner sole supports your foot's arch and leads the foot to the optimal position for pushing off.
At the same time it ensures that your center of gravity is lowered in the case of extreme instep (super-pronation). In this way you save energy for the subsequent rise. The exterior sole also has a tread that reduces the risk of slipping.

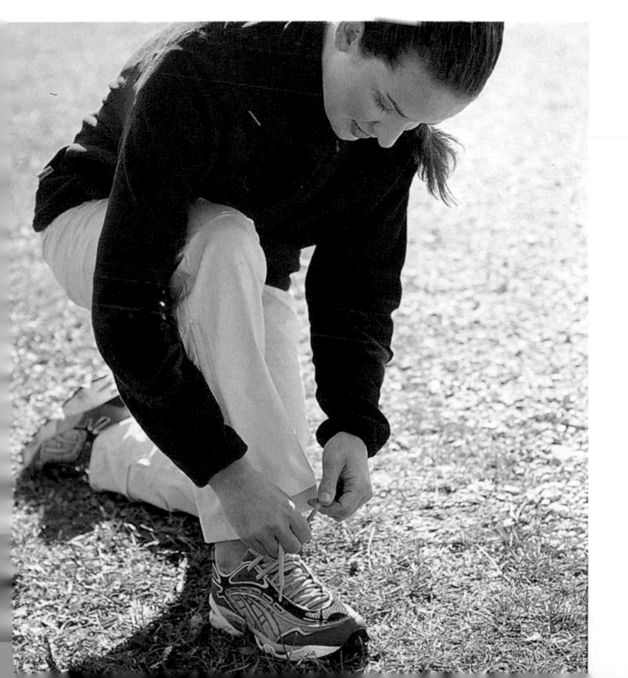

WALKING OR RUNNING SHOES?

INFO

For speed walking, walking on hard surfaces, or for anyone a little overweight, light running shoes that absorb shock well are ideal. Otherwise, you should use special speed walking shoes. These have more room in the front foot area as your toes spread more when speed walking than when running. Also, they have a slanted heel and a special middle sole to optimally support the foot's rolling motion.

Buying your shoes

In picking out your speed walking shoes the thing to pay attention to is whether the shoe fits your personal foot shape and motion. In specialized sporting goods stores your feet can be analyzed by video in two phases: at rest and while speed walking on a treadmill. A specialist can then recognize whether you walk with supination (an outward roll), pronation (inward roll), or straight.

The right size

Always buy speed walking shoes a little too big so that there is some room for your toes. During speed walking your feet will heat up and expand. This will result in pressure spots and painful blisters. As a rule, there should be a thumb's width of space in front of your big toe.
It's also a good idea to try the new shoes on with the socks you plan on wearing while walking.
Walk a few feet back and forth in the store or you might even ask to walk a short distance on the street with them. Make sure that your shoes fit comfortably on your heel and at the widest point of your foot and that your feet don't slide around in them.
If a shoe is too tight in any place, put it back on the shelf and try the next one!
There are also speed walking shoes available with watertight or water-resistant surfaces. This way you can keep your feet dry in any kind of weather.

CHECKLIST

KEEP IN MIND WHEN BUYING YOUR SHOES

- Give yourself enough time to try on various models.
- Buy your shoes in a specialty store, perhaps with a video analysis.
- Fit the shoes to your own personal foot shape.
- Always buy your shoes a little too large.
- Look for good shock absorbency in your shoes.

What foot type are you?

To determine your foot type quickly and definitively, several specialty stores offer a foot shape analysis. Your footprint will show by way of a special measuring plate whether you have normal, flat, splayed, or high-arched feet. You can also determine which foot type you are with a simple trick: Stand with wet feet on an absorbent surface, a piece of blotting paper for instance. To be sure, make a print with both feet.

Normal feet

The ball and middle of your foot as well as your heel are grouped together as connected parts. The area around your arch left no print. When running, a normal-footed person places his or her foot with the outer edge of the heel first and then turns it slightly inward as the foot unfurls. This guarantees good stability and an equalized shock absorbency. The ideal shoe for a normal-footed person is stable and has a slightly bowed edge, that is, the shoe's inner side is slightly bowed.

Flat or splayed feet

This foot type has a low and weak arch. For this reason the print (above right) shows almost the entire sole, an extreme instep whereby the foot is turned inward while walking heel-to-toe (superpronation). To compensate for this false positioning the proper shoes must offer this missing shock absorbency and stability. An arch support which is cushioned on the inside supports your arch and thus prevents your foot from turning too sharply while walking.

High-arched feet

In the case of high-arched feet, your arches are so high that the print shows nothing at all of the entire mid-section of your feet. When running, those with high arches touch the ground first with the outer midsection of their foot, which does not turn inward when unfurling. Because of this, there is a lack of shock protection and natural cushioning. The proper shoe must compensate for this and be especially shock absorbent and flexible. An arch support which is harder on the outside and softer on the inside is ideal.

The proper walking apparel

Always use functional clothing when running or speed walking. In contrast to cotton, microfibers do not absorb moisture – whether rain or sweat – but quickly release it again. Ideal clothing protects against wind and simultaneously aids in the release of surplus body heat. In this way functional running clothes act as a temperature regulator: excess heat evaporates for a cooling effect and your skin stays dry and comfortably warm.

CHECKLIST

SPEED WALKING APPAREL

- If you want to get some walking garments, you should buy: undergarments, shirts, and pants made from functional synthetic fibers, breathable and water-resistant rain gear, a cap, headband, and gloves.
- Always dress a little too cool to avoid unnecessary buildup of body heat.
- Wear clothes in several layers according to the onion principle.

Basic gear

When you first begin speed walking, you should equip yourself with the proper clothing. In the beginning it's enough to wear comfortable and airy clothing. Above all, do not dress too warmly because thick clothes can easily lead to a buildup of excess heat and thus to a rapid depletion of stamina. It's better to wear several layers, the so-called onion principle. Then you can relieve yourself of one layer after the other. Make sure that all materials will let your body breathe.

Specially for women

The answer to the question whether you should wear tight or loose pants when speed walking depends on your upper thighs. If your upper thighs rub against each other when walking, tight pants are better than loose ones, so that your sensitive skin is not irritated.
Another important point for women: regardless of whether you have a large or small bust, always wear a special sports bra. It supports your breasts and your sensitive tissue and prevents shaking. In the case of a small to medium bust, a bra without support cups is usually sufficient. If you have a larger bust, it is advisable to go for a bra with supports. The following

points are important when choosing your bra:

- The elastic support band should not be too loose but sit snug to your chest without constricting. It also should not rub. To check positioning, put your arm in the air and run in place. If the bra slips or is uncomfortable, this means it is not suitable.
- Buttons, zippers, or hooks should not press against your skin.
- Make sure there is sufficient elasticity and breathing room.

There is no such thing as bad weather.

Disregarding extreme weather conditions such as slick ice, you can equip yourself against cold or rain showers with the proper running clothes. Wear a wind- and rain resistant jacket that lets your body breathe as well in the case of wet, gray weather. A hood, a sweatband, or a cap helps against the loss of body heat. Remember, two-thirds of your body heat is released through your head. If your hands become uncomfortably cold, wear thin gloves equipped with a wind-breaking function. In the case of poor weather conditions such as fog or darkness, or in terrain with poor visibility, a reflective vest or a jacket with reflector stripes serves as a sufficient safety precaution.

Socks

If you have developed blisters, you should first check to see if your shoes are too small. If this is not the case, try training again with special running socks. They are seamless and cause less friction. Like the rest of the functional apparel, they also are constructed to let your feet breathe and whisk moisture away quickly.

Functional, breathable textiles will keep you comfortably warm even in winter.

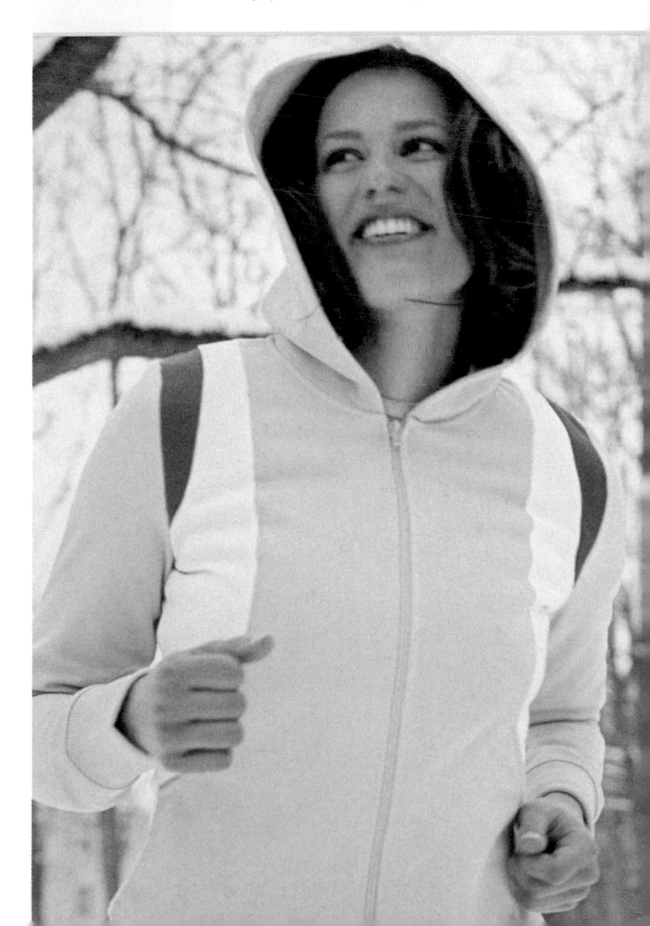

Devices for heart rate measurement

It is nearly impossible to manually measure your pulse rate while speed walking. In addition, your exercise pulse immediately slows down whenever you interrupt your walking. So, regardless of whether the slowdown is rapid or gradual, the results will always be inaccurate.

The chest belt for a pulse watch is worn in the area next to your heart.

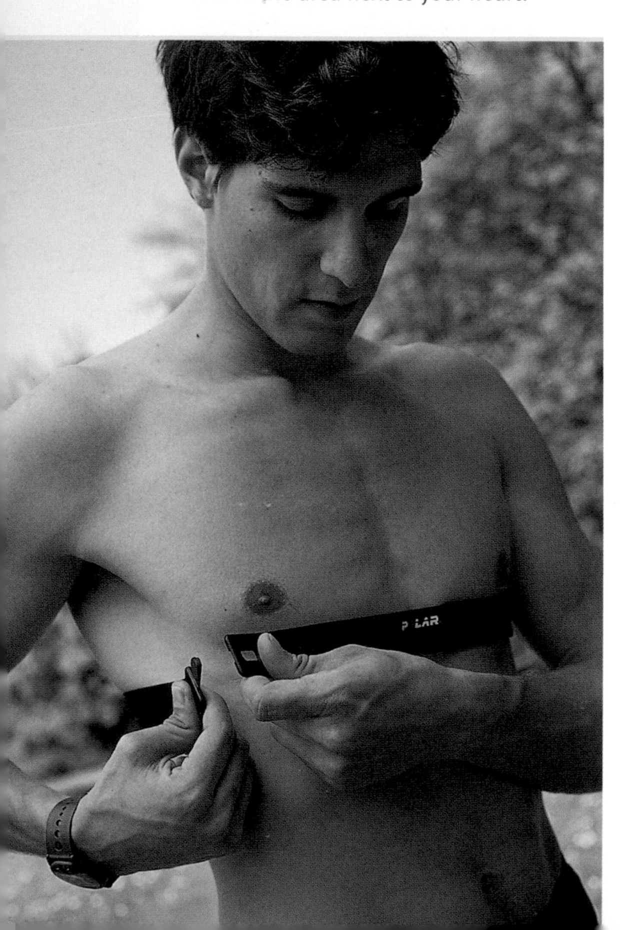

If you value exact pulse measurements you can use a heart rate/pulse monitor. A chest band wirelessly transmits the pulses your heart gives off every time it contracts, which are then received by the pulse watch.
You can read your heart rate and speed on the watch while walking and thus immediately increase or reduce your speed as soon as you exceed or drop below your training pulse rate. You can learn how high your optimal training pulse rate should be on page 49.

Technology's finest

With modern pulse watches you can program your training range before you begin, thereby determining your minimum and maximum pulse, which should be anywhere between 120 and 140. If you walk too slowly or too quickly, exceeding or dropping below this rate, then the watch will send an acoustic signal and you can change your tempo to meet the proper rate. Also integrated into almost all models are training length, time memory, and a stopwatch function.
The luxury models can even determine your own personal training range based on your form that day. Another monitor informs you of how many calories you're burning and how high your

fat burning ratio was. With these measuring devices you can even exclude the possibility of signal interruption from other power walkers, such as when city walking.

It's better with music

Music invigorates and helps many people to switch out of their everyday routine and tank up on new energy – when power walking too. If you find it difficult to motivate yourself for training, you should try it once with musical accompaniment. The rhythm will help you forget the exertion. Also, a portable CD player or walkman with headphones hardly adds to your total weight load.
Which music you pick out depends of course on your own personal taste – whichever CD you favor at the moment is always good. The musical rhythm also develops its own dynamic and has an influence on your walking tempo. Pop, new age, and light jazz are ideal for power walking beginners who are training at a low pulse rate. Lively Latin rhythms on the other hand will add some additional heat to your training session and stimulate your motivational stamina. There are even special speed walking CDs in many specialty stores offering music for beginners, advanced walkers, and experts – some with slower, others with faster pieces.

Speed walking with weights?

Be careful when speed walking with additional weights on your arms. Your motion may change through the increased load, which may lead to muscle strain in your shoulders and neck. If you really do want to try it, then at least do so without dumbbells! These lead to cramped hand posture and increase circulatory disturbances. Wear weighted wristbands instead. 3.5 to 7 ounces suffice as the weight compounds at a terrific rate: if you walk for one hour with a 7-ounce weight, you will be carrying the equivalent of an additional three tons at 120 movements per arm.

Alternatives to weights

If you want to do something for your arms, Nordic walking might be an option (see page 78). Walking with sticks entails an ideal arm training because of the constant arm motion. With a specific power workout for your arms (page 102) you can support your walking program another way.

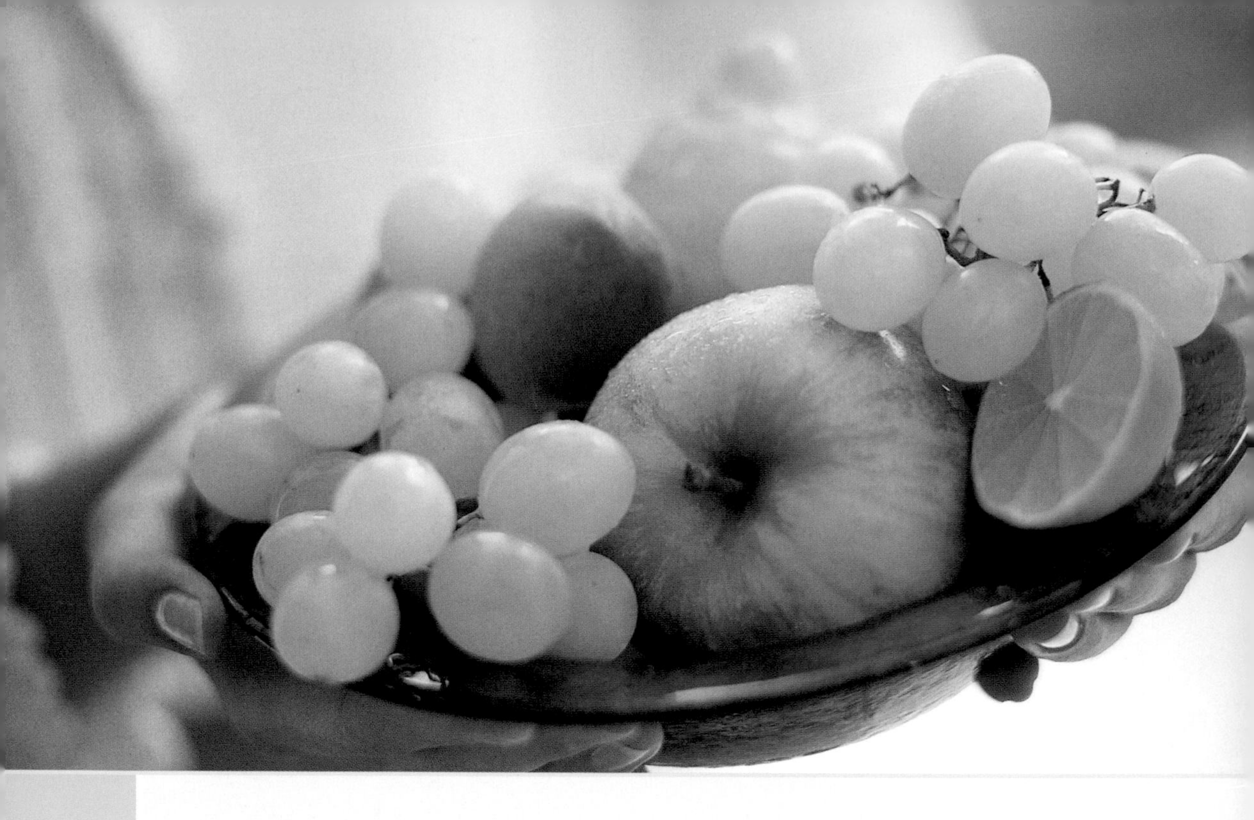

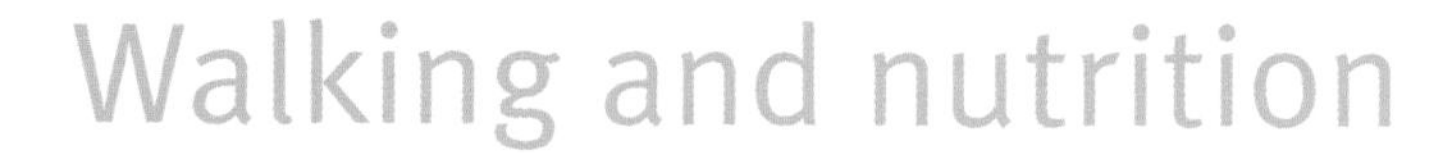

Walking and nutrition

If you want to lose weight in the long term, there's no way of getting around regular endurance training. If you exercise, you burn calories. But this alone will not suffice. One of the most popular nutrition myths is that you can eat whatever you want as long as you exercise enough. The truth is: You have to strike the proper balance. If you consume more energy (calories) than you burn, you will gain weight. And only when you start burning more calories than you consume will the pounds begin to melt away.

However, not all people are fighting against being overweight. Even if you are actually completely satisfied with your figure, a balanced, nutritional diet will help you stay healthy, increase your stamina, and maintain the body weight you feel most comfortable with.

In addition you should follow some nutrition rules with walking – as with all sports.

No more dieting

A lot of people have tried one or more crash diets at least once – "15 pounds in one week" and similar promises simply sound too alluring. Indeed, in the beginning you will usually lose weight quite quickly, especially if it's just water that your body is getting rid of at the time. But most people don't care! After all, the scale goes down, and that is what motivates you to keep it up. But as soon as you're eating "normally" again, your weight skyrockets and in very little time you weigh even more than before you started the diet.

The yo-yo effect

Behind the fact that we regain the pounds lost when dieting at an abnormal rate lies a genetic (emergency) program that has been hardwired into our bodies for millennia. The reason is that as soon as your body begins receiving nourishment in insufficient quantities it switches over to standby to compensate for the calorie deficit. The result: you stop losing weight! Now, if you start eating again like you did before the diet, your body attempts to lock as much energy in its reserves as possible to be equipped for the next "state of emergency". It then requires a larger energy supply and more nourishment, and this is why you gain a few more pounds.

Only skinny without dieting

To counteract the yo-yo effect, you have to forget the idea that you can only lose weight in the long term through a reduced calorie intake. What promises much more success is to completely change the foods you eat: plenty of fruit and vegetables, complex carbohydrates, high-quality protein, and essential fats should make up the bulk of your diet. If you then exercise more than you used to, you are guaranteed to lose weight!

IMPORTANT !

CAUTION: CRASH DIET

You consume too few calories with a crash diet. Your body will then take the missing energy out of the protein in your muscles instead of from fat cells. In this way your muscle mass will shrink and your basal metabolic rate sink. If you eat normally again after the diet, you will gain weight faster for this very reason.

Carbohydrates

Carbohydrates are the most important energy suppliers. They consist of diverse sugar building blocks that your body converts to glucose and burns directly as energy. If you speed walk often or are active in another endurance sport, carbohydrates should form the foundation of your diet, that is, at least 55 percent.
To put it simply, carbohydrates increase your stamina. Only if the carbohydrate reserves in your muscles and liver are well supplied can you exert yourself over a longer period and train with more intensity.

"Good" and "bad" carbohydrates

Not all carbohydrates are equally nutritious. Simple single and double carbohydrates such as sugar, white flour products, and white rice shoot straight into your blood and cause the blood sugar level to rise immediately. Your body then distributes increased levels of the hormone insulin to very quickly transport the sugar out of your bloodstream and into your cells. As a result, your blood sugar level sinks rapidly, causing your body to mistakenly desire new sugar.
A ravenous appetite is the result! If you then reach for more simple carbohydrates you will gain weight quickly – these foods are also usually combined with fat. Metabolizing complex carbohydrates such as whole grain foods, potatoes, and legumes, on the other hand, requires much more time. This means that the sugar flows into the bloodstream in increments and your blood sugar level rises less sharply and sinks again more evenly.

The Glycemic Index

The GLYX – an abbreviation for the glycemic index – is a measurement to determine how high insulin output is after consumption of a specific food type. In choosing carbohydrates, an endurance athlete should pick foods with a medium to low GLYX. In the case of a GLYX between 70 and 100, the insulin reaction is extremely high. For this reason you should abstain from eating these foods whenever possible and make sure, above all, that you do not combine them with fats. Fruit, vegetables and legumes almost always have a low GLYX (some exceptions are watermelons, cooked carrots, and squash or pumpkin).
Also, milk and dairy products can best be enjoyed without guilt in their low-fat or skim versions as they otherwise contain too much hidden fat. The same is true of meat, poultry, and fish.

INFO

GLYX – THE NUTRITION CHART

	Higher GLYX >70	Median GLYX 70–51	Low GLYX <51
Baked goods			
	pretzels	brown bread	whole barley bread
	croissants	pita bread	oat bread
	hamburger buns	pizza	multigrain bread
	crackers	pizza crust	pumpernickel
	rye bread	taco shells	soy bread with flax seed
	white bread	whole wheat crackers	whole wheat bread
Grains			
	cornflakes	basmati rice	brown rice
	müsli with sugar	couscous	noodles/bulgur
	puffed rice	white grits	oatmeal
	short-grain	white rice long-grain	whole grain müsli without sugar
Potatoes and pasta			
	roasted potatoes	gnocchi	cellophane mung bean noodles
	potato chips	raw potato dumplings	whole grain noodles
	mashed potatoes	semolina noodles	potato soup
	french fries	new potatoes	ravioli
	potato croquettes	baked potatoes	whole grain pasta
Sweets and snacks			
	ice cream	jam and jelly	dark chocolate (over 70% cocoa)
	gummy bears	oatcakes	fruit sorbet
	cake	honey	chewing gum
	chips	popcorn	baked apple with nuts
	chocolate	shortbread	granola bars with honey

Protein

Your body requires protein for the production of muscle mass. Non-professional athletes generally get a sufficient amount from the average, protein-rich diet. The important thing, though, is that this protein comes from low-fat foods, from lean meat, fish, eggs, low-fat milk, rice, oats, millet, and legumes. To ensure the optimal supply of various protein building blocks you should combine as many of these foods as possible. Something good to know: Protein has, of all nutrients, the highest capacity to fill you up. Besides this, it is also considered a so-called fat-burner and can really boost weight loss.

IMPORTANT !

SPEED WALKING ON A FULL STOMACH?

Wait for one to two hours after eating before you begin your training. A large quantity of blood is necessary for digestion, which takes it away from the oxygen supply to the muscles. This leads to side pains. Neither should you speed walk on an empty stomach. A banana or slice of whole grain bread is ideal as a pre-training snack.

Fat

One thing is clear: We eat too much fat! 140 grams of fat a day is no rarity these days. This is fatal, because half of this is plenty. If you want to lose weight you should only eat 30 to 40 grams of fat a day. On the other hand, to permanently abstain from any fat in your diet can be life-threatening, as your body cannot produce all the fatty acids on its own. The result: Your metabolism, hormonal balance, and digestion will not function. Besides, fat-soluble vitamins could not be integrated into your body.
It's not just a matter of quantity, but of which kind of fat you choose to eat:

- Saturated fatty acids from milk and dairy products, meat, sausage, sweets, cakes and pastries, and also palm and coconut fat raise cholesterol and increase the risk of arteriosclerosis because they build up on your blood vessel walls.
- Vegetable oils, fish, and nuts contain unsaturated, so-called Omega-3 fatty acids that are vital and protect against heart attacks, among other things. Particular protective are olive and rapeseed oils. These contain simple, unsaturated fatty acids.

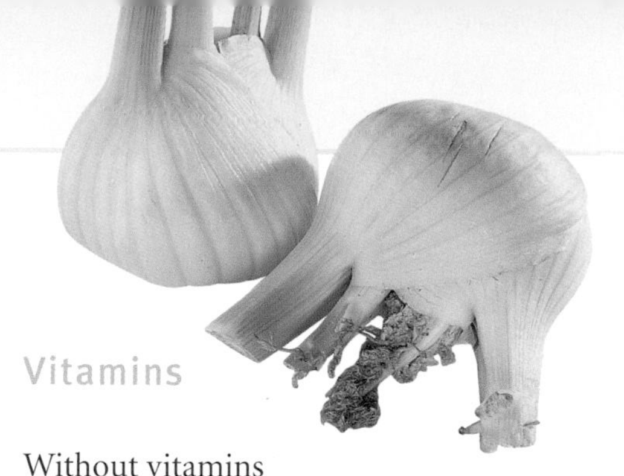

Vitamins

Without vitamins nothing would work to metabolize carbohydrates, proteins, and fats. Besides, they provide an important protection against "free radicals" – aggressive oxygen molecules in your cells which, among other things, speed up the aging process.
You have to consume almost all vitamins through your food because your body does not produce them itself. Fat-soluble vitamins (A, D, E, and K) can be stored by your body over a longer period. Water-soluble vitamins, on the other hand, (vitamins in the B group and vitamin C) must be consumed daily. This is only possible with a balanced and wholesome diet.

Minerals and trace elements

Vitamins can develop their full function only in combination with minerals and trace elements. If you are stressed or over-burdened, the risk is greater that too many minerals will be lost. Proper nutrition is especially important in this case. This is also true if you are active in many sports and physically exert yourself to a high degree. The most valuable sources of minerals are raw or lightly steamed vegetables, and mineral water (pay attention to the nutrition information on the label).
If you are physically active, many minerals and trace elements are excreted through sweat, making it necessary for you to replace these through proper nutrition. Especially important then are vitamins of the B group, vitamin C, folic acid, iron, magnesium, and zinc.

Secondary plant matter

Secondary plant matter refers to all substances in fruit and vegetables responsible for taste, smell, and appearance. Even if they are not counted among the vital nutrients like vitamins, they still have a certain value for our health and well-being that should not be underestimated. When boiled, baked, or otherwise cooked, this sensitive organic matter is lost just as it is through the overly long storage of food. One more reason to serve fruit and vegetables as fresh as possible, and raw!

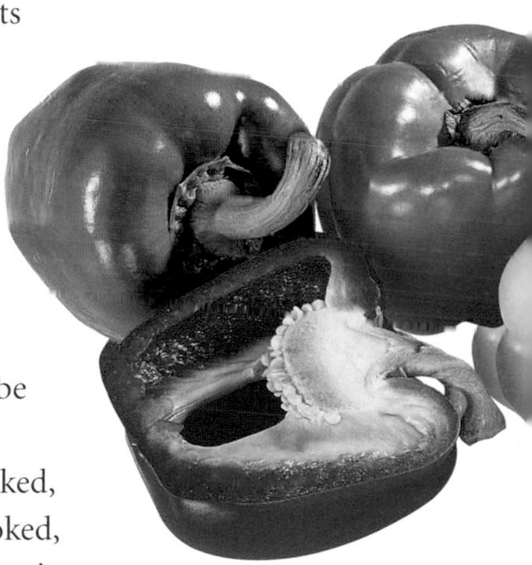

Fiber

Fiber makes you full because it wells up in your body. It keeps your intestinal flora alive and detoxifies your body by quickly removing damaging substances from your digestive tract.
Just three slices of whole grain bread, two apples, and three carrots are enough to fulfill a daily fiber requirement of around 30 grams. If you eat fruit and vegetables, you don't just consume a lot of fiber, you simultaneously consume plentiful vitamins, minerals, and secondary plant matter – and only for a few calories in exchange!

Keeping hydrated

We can survive for a few weeks without eating with no problem, but not even three days without water. Cooling moisture is truly an elixir of life. No wonder then that we ourselves consist of 60 to 70 percent water. To feel healthy and fit you have to drink at least four pints of water a day – evenly distributed, because your body cannot absorb more than one and a half pints an hour. And for each half-hour of exercise per day you must also drink one pint of fluid extra.

The best thirst quencher

Cover your daily requirement of fluid with mineral or simple tap water, sparkling fruit spritzers (in the ratio of one part juice to one part water), or unsweetened fruit or herbal tea. Coffee and black tea on the other hand are pleasure drinks that you cannot count as part of your daily ration and actually contribute to an increase in fluid loss. For this reason you should drink one extra glass of water for each cup of coffee.

TIP

CAUTION: CALORIE BOMB!

Hands off soda pop, sweetened juices, and other soft drinks! They have a lot of calories and contain ridiculous amounts of sugar, which goes straight into your bloodstream. Alcohol also has almost as many calories as fat: seven kilocalories per gram.

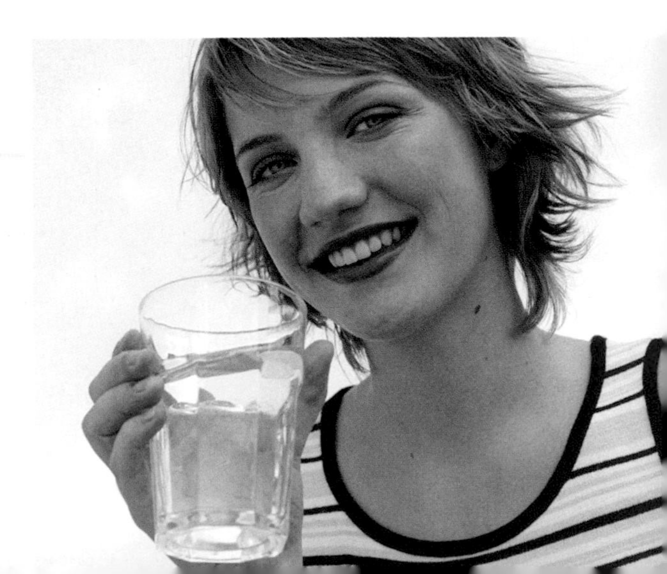

DOES YOUR BODY NEED MORE ENERGY NOW?

I have heard that the body takes its energy from fat when speed walking at a slow pace. Does it need more fat then?

It's true that your body, when training in the so-called fat-burning zone (60 to 70 percent of the maximum pulse rate) gets the majority of the energy it requires from its own fat deposits. These, however, are sufficiently full even in thin people. 30 to 40 grams of fat in your daily diet, best from olive or rapeseed oil, are really enough to provide your body with vital fatty acids.

I have heard that it's better to eat several times throughout the day than to eat three large meals. Is it true?

That depends! The advantage of it is that your blood sugar level remains relatively constant throughout the day and you are spared any ravenous hunger. But for many people, six or seven small snacks quickly become six or seven large meals. Especially people with weight problems will not notice when they become full. They eat until the plate or the package is empty and consume in this way far too many calories.

Do food supplements promote speed walking stamina?

If you choose to believe the scientists, the use of food supplements makes sense for certain high-risk groups such as pregnant women. Protein or carbohydrate concentrates can also have a positive effect on muscle growth and athletic stamina for serious athletes. As a hobby athlete, however, you can easily do without food supplements. Instead, try to eat a balanced diet: 55 to 60 percent of your daily nourishment should be covered by valuable carbohydrates, 10 to 15 percent by protein, and around 25 to 30 percent by fat. And discuss any possible nutrition eficiencies with your doctor before reaching for food supplements.

I don't think that I eat too much. Despite this, I'm still gaining weight. How can that be?

Keep a nutritional journal in which you write down everything you eat each day. Don't forget that piece of chocolate or the handful of nuts between meals either. Only this way can you objectively monitor where your weak points are and then make any changes.

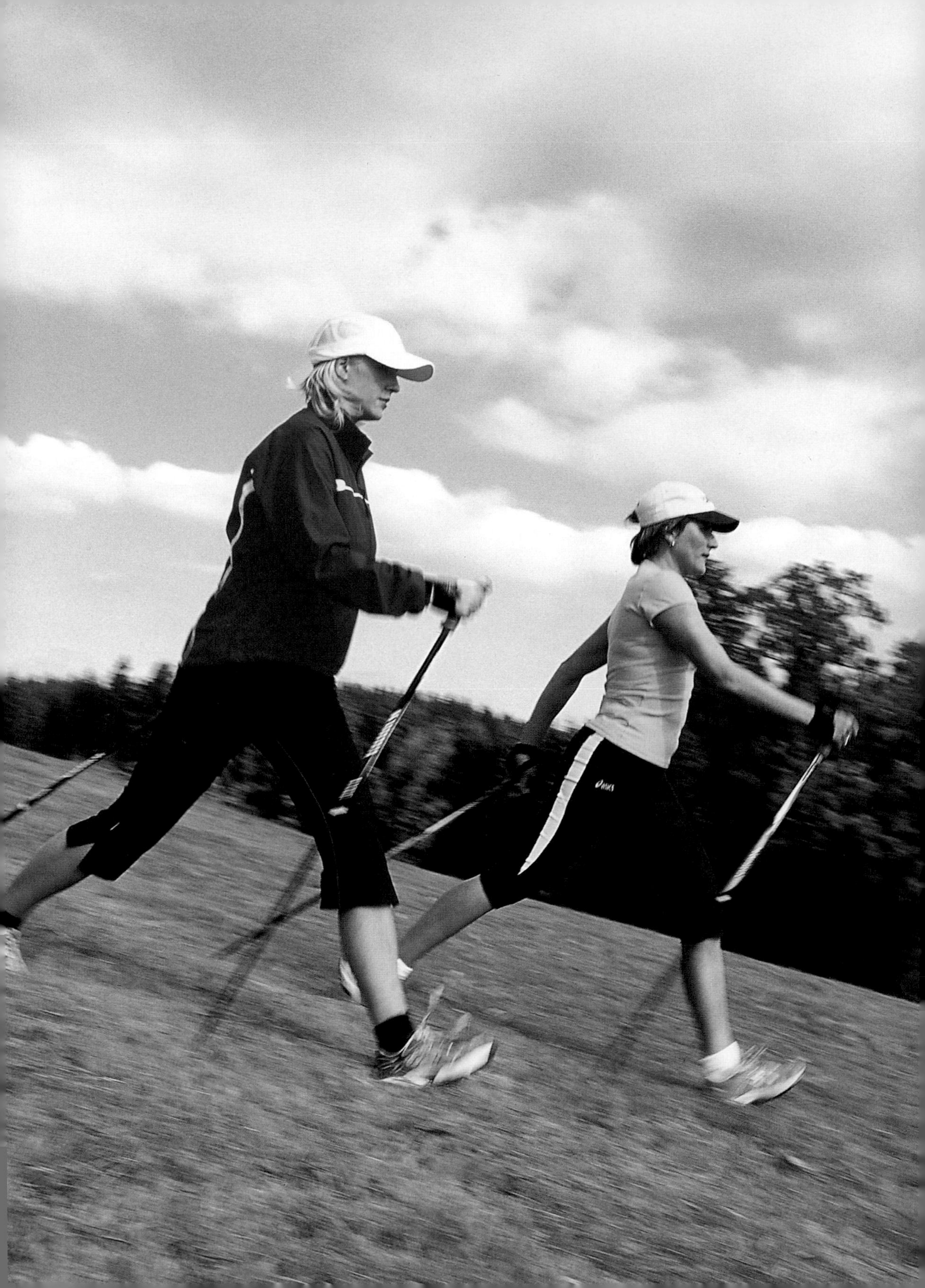

Walking for experts

Walking has a great deal more to offer those looking for a challenge in their training. You can speed up your tempo with power walking and boost your circulation, or try Nordic walking, which promotes whole-body exercise. With light running you can even let your feet leave the ground briefly: quick running phases thus alternate with milder walking periods.

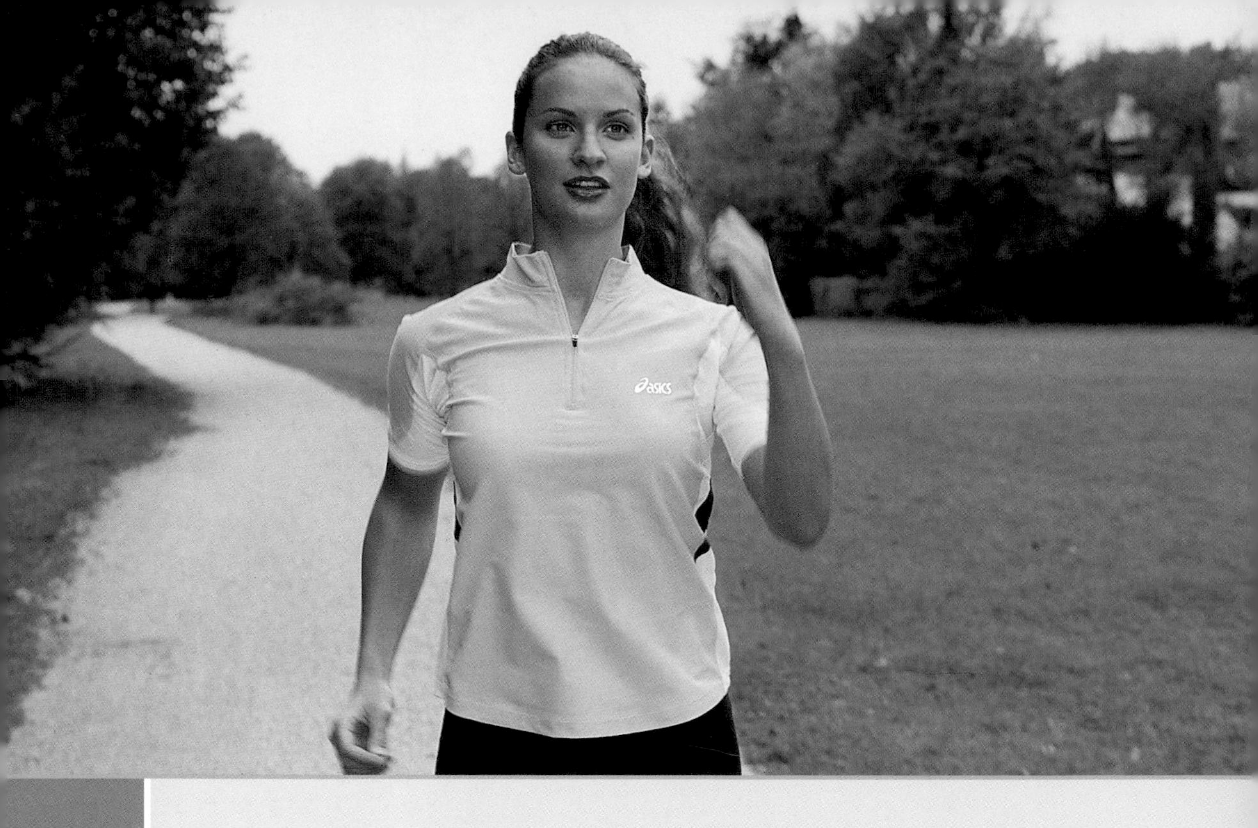

Power walking

Power walking is exactly the right thing for you if you received result A in the Stamina checkup on page 20. This faster variant of speed walking is, to use a turn of phrase, the "Formula 1" of speed walking and for this reason is the ideal program for ambitious and well-conditioned walkers. With power or "fitness" walking you walk at the highest possible speed without crossing over into the Olympic competition "walking". Your heart rate increases with the higher speed, which has a positive effect on your circulatory system in particular. Power walking is cardio-vascular training in which the training pulse rate rises to 75 or 80 percent. At the same time, this variant is very well-suited to overcoming training stagnation and increasing stamina. The reason for this is that your body must draw on energy reserves when it becomes subjected to greater demands.

Get some speed!

The faster you walk, the quicker mistakes can creep up to you. So pay special attention to proper walking technique. You should begin – even if you're fit – with a few minutes of slow walking. At this time you can still concentrate on the unfurling of your feet and active arm motion.
If you let yourself go at full speed there is always the danger that your movements will become too haphazard. Your speed walking program would not have its desired effect then.
In the worst case scenario, the wrong movements could even lead to muscular disorders or problems with your shoulders or back.

Walking faster made easy

The easiest way to increase your speed is to move your arms more quickly. Follow this motto: Your arms determine your speed, and your feet and legs will follow!
Also pay attention to the proper arm movements: Swing your arms from the side of your body and do not cross them in front of your body. Also, your elbows should not swing any higher than your breastbone. Otherwise too much energy is wasted.

Time to regenerate

If you train harder your body requires more breaks for its own regeneration. To take full advantage of your power potential you should go two days between training sessions to let your body recover from the increased exertion demanded of it.

Power walking rules

- Make sure your steps are not too big! Otherwise you will interrupt your forward motion – which costs unnecessary energy.

TIP

INTERVAL TRAINING

If you want to just try out power walking for the first time or don't think that you're fit enough to maintain your maximum speed over a longer stretch, go ahead and try what's called interval training. With interval training, slower and faster walking phases alternate within a single training session. Shorten the slower phases more and more until you are at last able to walk the whole stretch at a power walking speed.

- Move your arms rhythmically, but not too energetically.
- Don't look at the ground but rather four or five yards ahead.
- Don't raise up your shoulders. Instead, let them relax and hang slightly back and under.
- Do not carry any weights so that no false movements occur.

Training program for power walking

With this program it's not hard to achieve your desired training load and training speed. Nevertheless, begin slowly and increase at a constant rate so that you don't lose any of your motivation.

Weeks 1 to 4

Start your training with three sessions per week. Walk on level or only slightly sloping terrain. You still should not walk too far or too fast right away.
30 to 45 minutes per session with a heart rate of 60 to 75 percent (page 49) is plenty.

Weeks 5 to 8

Increase your performance. Your heart rate should already be around 75 percent in this week without you running out of breath to reach this figure. Training length increases to 45 to 60 minutes, three to four times a week.

Weeks 9 to 12

60 minutes at a time (and more) with a training pulse rate of around 80 percent is no problem for you anymore.
To prevent the stamina you've achieved from subsiding, continue walking three to four times a week. Your condition is already so good that you can plan a small mountain jog into your training. This will provide some variety.

INFO

TRAINING PROGRAM POWER WALKING

Weeks	1–4	5–8	9–12
Optimal Heart Rate (% of max. pulse)	60–75 %	75 %	75–80 %
Training Time per Session (in minutes)	30–45	45–60	60 +
Sessions per Week	3	3–4	3–4

FINDING THE RIGHT LEVEL

I enjoy walking with friends. But, even though we all train at about the same speed, my pulse rate is around ten percent higher than the others. Does that mean I'm less fit?

Pulse rate is an individual measurement that depends on various criteria such as age, gender, strength, and stamina. So, as a general rule, it's completely normal for your figures to diverge from each other within a certain range.
Still, you should make sure that you're not training in the anaerobic range and completely exhausting yourself. If your friends set too high a speed, you should address the problem or perhaps it's better for you to train on your own. Otherwise, you will soon find yourself training as if for a competitive sport – and the fun and motivation will quickly be lost.

A girlfriend bought herself special women's running shoes. Does that really contribute something to your training?

Yes, because women's feet are usually slimmer, higher in the instep, and broader at the toes and heel than men's feet. Also, the ankle joint is positioned higher with women than with men. So, good women's shoes are not just smaller versions of men's shoes but are constructed to meet the special needs of their foot.
Very important: Do not buy your shoes too small, otherwise you'll get blisters!

I started power walking a few weeks ago and would like to train every day. Is it true that your body needs breaks in between, or can I follow my urges for more exercise?

Less is more! In regards to performance, days of rest are extremely important, especially because hobby athletes enjoy running too fast and over-exert themselves this way (often without noticing it). You should not forego those long periods of recuperation. If you feel the pull of the outdoors so much, go for an energetic stroll for about an hour on your training-free days. You also tank up on fresh air and get spiritual relief this way.

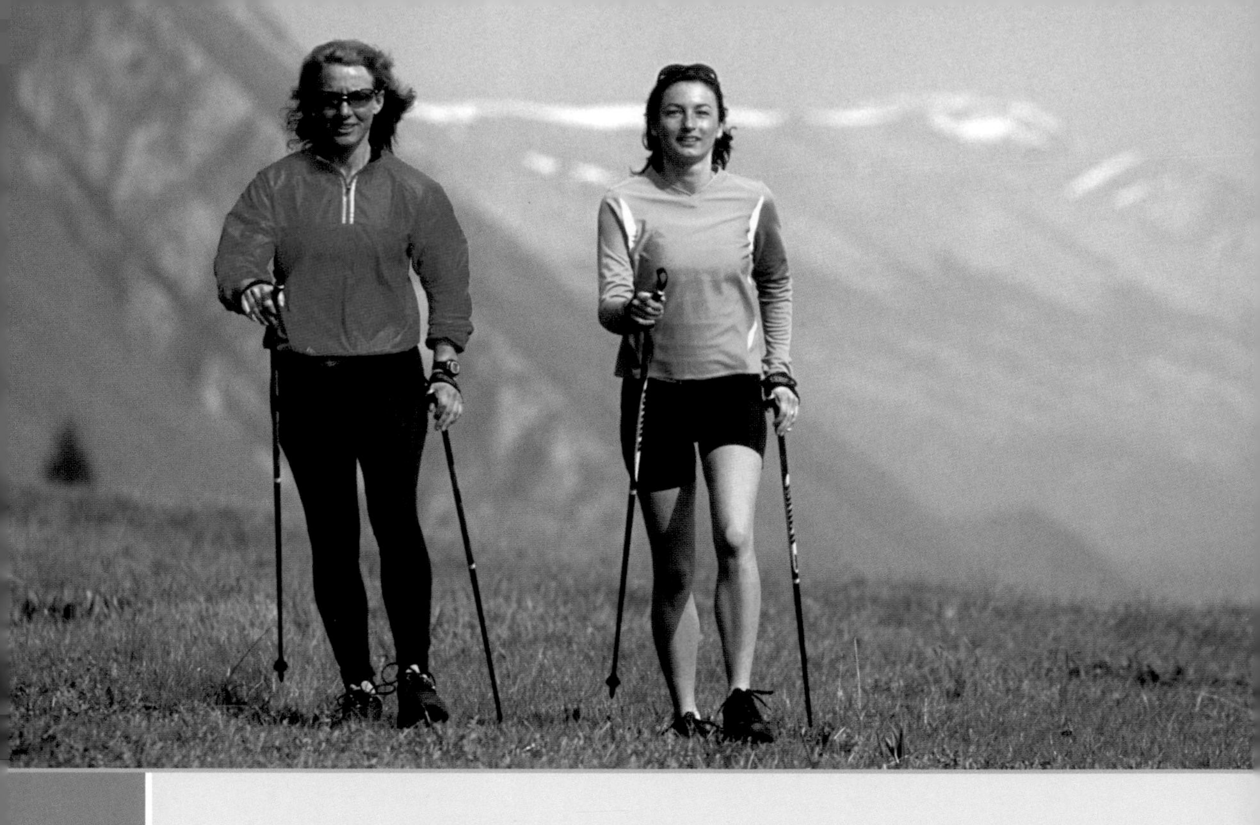

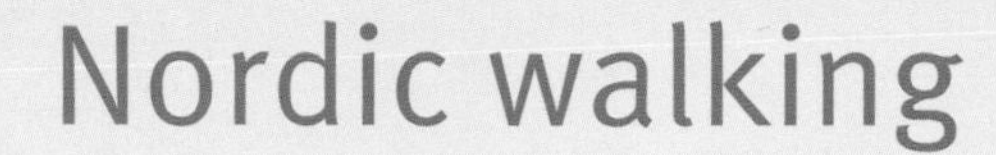

Nordic walking

This walking trend originated in Finland and is called Nordic walking. It was originally conceived as a summer training for cross-country skiers and biathletes. Nordic walking has long been a beloved common sport in the far north. In the Alpine region as well there are also great many supporters of this speed walking variant. So, it's only a question of time before Nordic walking spreads to the USA and other countries. The Finnish version's peculiar element is the use of special walking sticks. This is why hecklers sometimes call Nordic walking "cross country skiing without the snow". But what might at first sight appear unusual is an advantage in the eyes of speed walkers! The special sticks promote not only an especially active use of your arms – a true fitness plus! – but also give you a hold when walking on uneven terrain and allow for year-round training, even in snow and ice.

Healthy whole-body training

Nordic walking has more advantages to offer from a health and athletic perspective. Nordic walking is an especially effective whole-body training method. Because of the active integration of walking sticks, not only are your legs and rear being toned but the muscles in your shoulder area, back, chest, and arms are decidedly strengthened. This is ideal for women who would like to do more for these parts of their body without going into a gym. Additionally, you can train for greater power if you walk uphill Working with walking sticks has yet another considerable advantage from health perspective: The walking sticks provide an almost automatic correction in your posture, which in turn ensures optimal oxygen consumption. The oxygen content in your bloodstream increases by as much as 50 percent and your cardiovascular performance is boosted.

Relief for your joints

Like power walking, Nordic walking intensifies your normal training – and in a particularly easy manner for your joints. The entire passive system of mobility, that is, your tendons and ligaments, as well as your back and joints (especially your knees) are relieved just through the use of walking sticks – at a rough estimate by around 15 to 35 tons each hour. For this reason Nordic walking is ideal as a rehabilitation sport for anyone suffering from orthopedic issues. In Scandinavia, Nordic walking is used as a means of therapy in numerous physical therapy clinics, and in Germany some health insurance companies are already investing in Nordic walking courses as part of their preventive programs.

Losing weight with nordic walking

Not only do walkers with previous musculoskeletal complaints profit from the relief offered by the accompanying walking sticks, those with weight problems do as well. After all, each extra pound signifies an increased strain on your joints and tendons. And a further plus: By utilizing more muscles, your entire energy consumption increases. Because of the increase in oxygen intake, fat burning is also boosted. In numbers this means, compared to normal speed walking, you burn more calories with Nordic walking – in one hour you burn around 400. If you're losing weight and want to maintain your figure over the long term, Nordic walking is the optimal endurance sport for you.

Working off stress effectively

Just like normal speed walking, Nordic walking also helps you work off everyday stress and psychological pressures through exercise in the open air. Tension in the shoulder and neck area is also relieved by the intensive use of walking poles; this is especially helpful for people who are plagued by such tension after sitting most of the day at a desk.
Unlike speed walking with weights (see page 63), walking with poles does not lead to haphazard arm movement and tense shoulders. On the contrary, your muscles relax with each step and pole movement!
Back pain – a frequent symptom of stress and psychological overload – is also reduced through regular Nordic walking.

INFO

THE ADVANTAGES OF NORDIC WALKING

- Increases oxygen intake.
- Boosts your cardiovascular performance.
- You burn more calories than with normal speed walking because of the use of poles.
- Tension in your neck and shoulders dissolves.
- You build muscle in your legs, rear, chest, back, and arms.
- Sure-footed training also on uneven terrain.

Equipment

You generally require the same gear for Nordic walking as you do for regular speed walking (see page 56). Once again, the important thing is having proper shoes and, of course, poles.

The right shoes

In contrast to regular speed walking, you take longer steps when Nordic walking. Also, you train less in the park and on the street then you do in true outdoor terrain. This is also something to keep in mind when buying your shoes. The proper shoes should have especially good traction with anti-skidding soles and good shock absorbency. They must support your feet in every phase of motion as well as be extremely weather-resistant. In any case, you should try on different models to determine which one optimally conforms to your feet. Walk around inside and, better yet, outside the shop for a sufficient amount of time. You can find more tips about buying shoes on page 58.

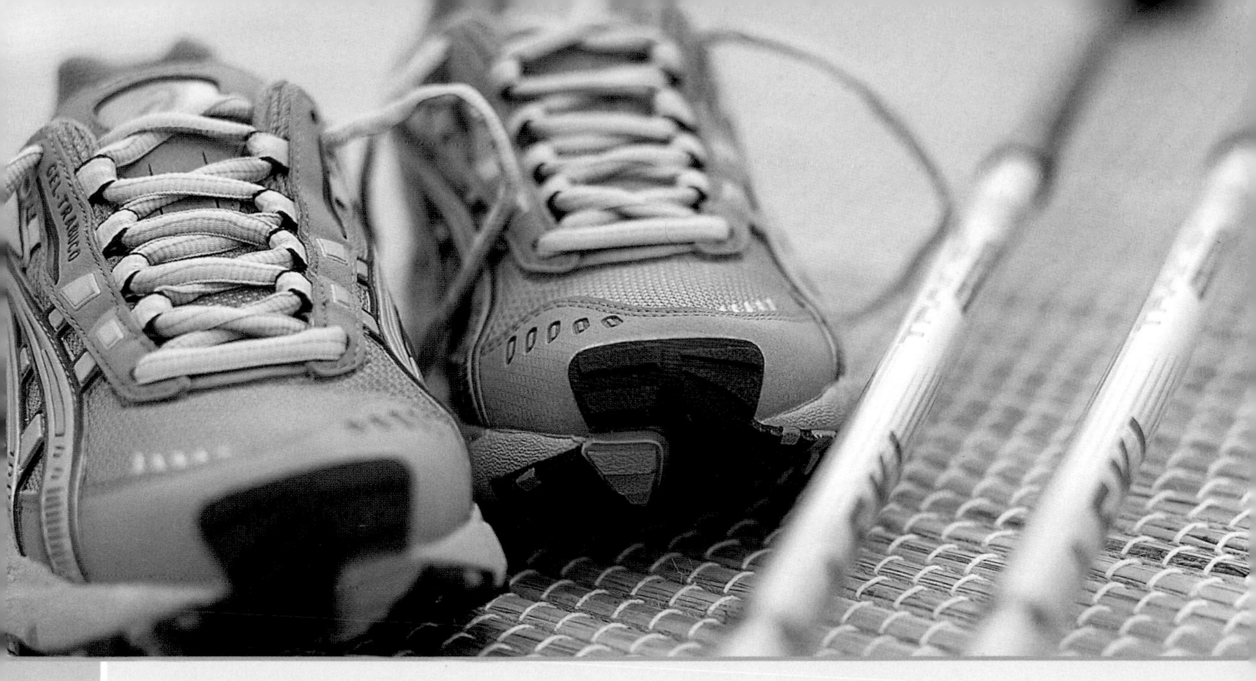

In addition to good shoes you also need special walking poles for Nordic walking.

Walking sticks

Nordic walking sticks, or poles, can be bought in any specialty sports shop these days. They're longer than the usual walking sticks for hikers and have well-designed handgrips and metal points just like cross-country ski poles. They offer protection against stumbling even when walking on rough terrain or slippery ice, and are therefore the perfect prerequisite for year-round training. In contrast to other walking sticks, Nordic walking poles have special hand straps so that your hands can open during backswing, a design which prevents muscle pain. When buying your poles, make sure that the straps have velcro closures so that they can be fitted to your individual hand shape and easily secured.

There are fine but important differences when it comes to the materials used. Poles constructed from a fiberglass mixture have the advantage over those with a metal core in that they do not transfer burdensome shocks to your wrists, elbows, or shoulders. If you walk on asphalt it is advisable to put a rubber cap on the metal points of your poles (you can find these in sports shops). The most important thing when it comes to your poles, besides a robust construction, is the correct length, which depends on your own height. The formula for determining the optimal pole length in inches is the following: height in feet x 7.8. You can find walking poles in increments of two inches. Experienced walkers use poles that are two to four inches longer than the normal size (see the box on page 82).

Technique

Like speed walking, Nordic walking is quite easy to pick up. But there are a few small differences:

- The pace length increases.
- Arm use decreases.
- Your whole body is utilized with greater strength.

If you follow the instructions below, the technique will doubtless become second nature in no time.

Beginning posture

- Let your shoulders hang loose and relaxed.
- Hold the poles close to your body.

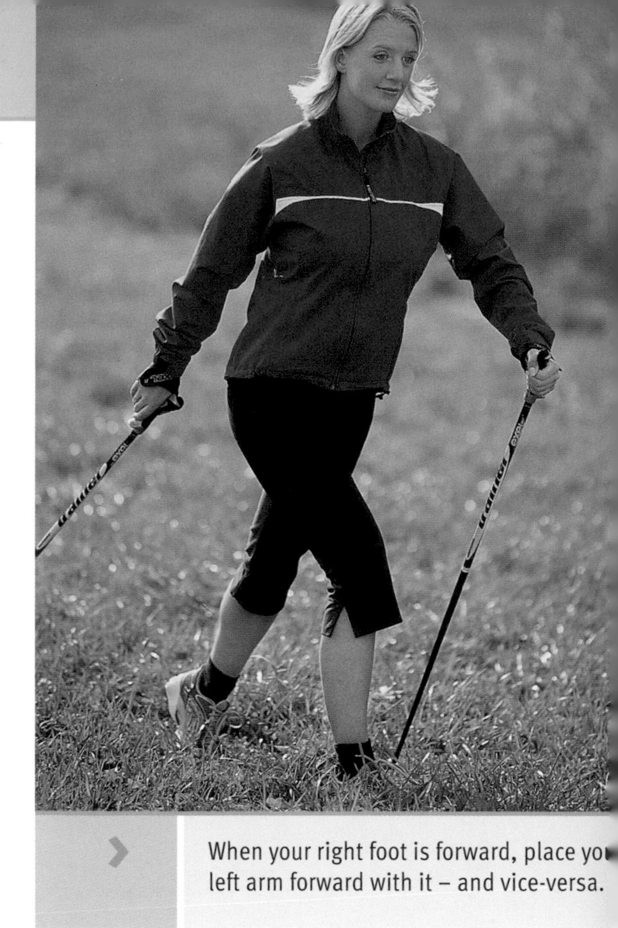

When your right foot is forward, place your left arm forward with it – and vice-versa.

INFO

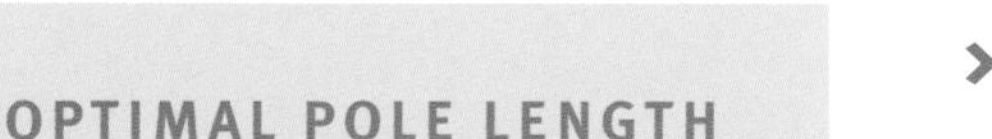

OPTIMAL POLE LENGTH

Height in feet/inches	**Pole Length** in inches
6' 56"	51
6' 40"	51
6' 24"	49
6' 70"	47
5' 91"	47
5' 75"	45
5' 58"	43
5' 42"	43
5' 25"	41

- Keep your hands slightly open to allow the poles to swing.
- Point your feet forward.

Let's go!

- Stand on your left leg with your knee slightly bent. Stretch your right leg out behind you. Stretch your right arm out in front of you, elbow bent. The right pole's metal point should be positioned at the height of your left heel. Your left arm should stretch out behind you. Keep your hand open. The pole serves as an extension of your arm.

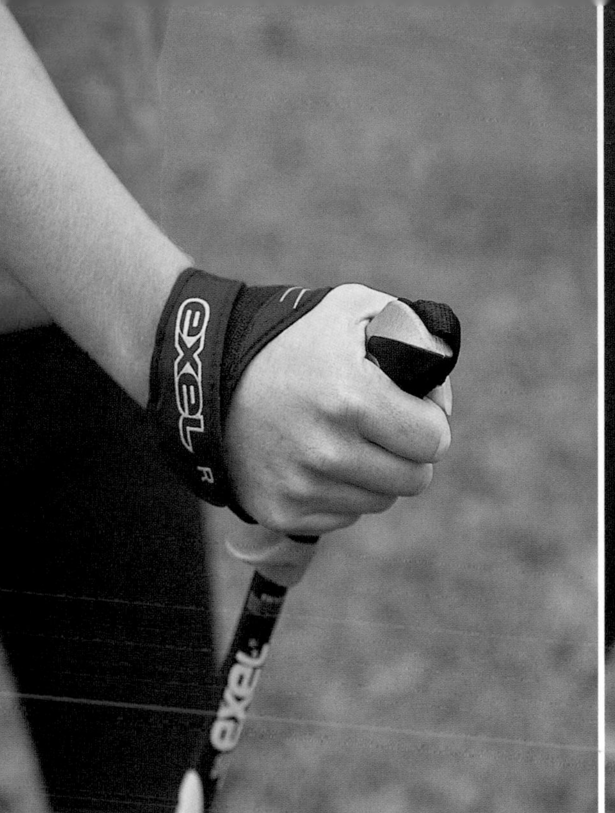

Each pole should be placed at heel height. Push off with closed hands.

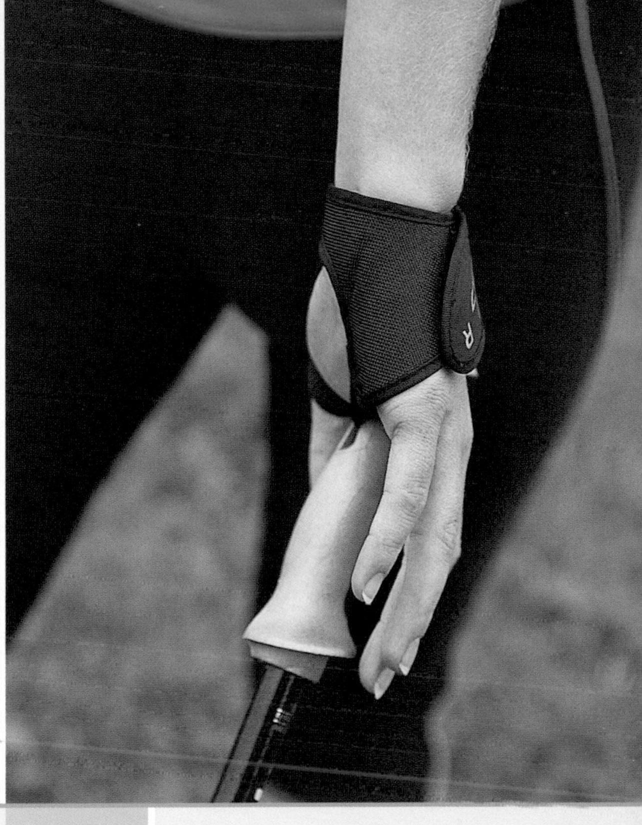

The pole should loosely swing backwards. Keep your hand open.

- Your right leg and left arm move forward. Set your right heel down and place the left pole's metal point at the same height as your right heel.
- Roll your foot forward and support yourself vigorously with the use of the left pole. Your left leg and right arm should be stretched out behind you. Keep your hand open and hold the pole as if an extension of your own arm.
- This way, your left leg and right arm, and your right leg and left arm alternate their movements backwards and forwards in a rhythmic manner.

Proper placement of foot and pole

Your walking poles should point backwards at an angle the whole time you're walking. The points of the poles are never positioned in front of your body. Keep the poles close to your body and let your arms hang loosely. Your elbows should never be too sharply angled and your poles never placed in front of your body. Make sure that your right foot and left pole, and left foot and right pole remain active. The correct posture will then come almost automatically.

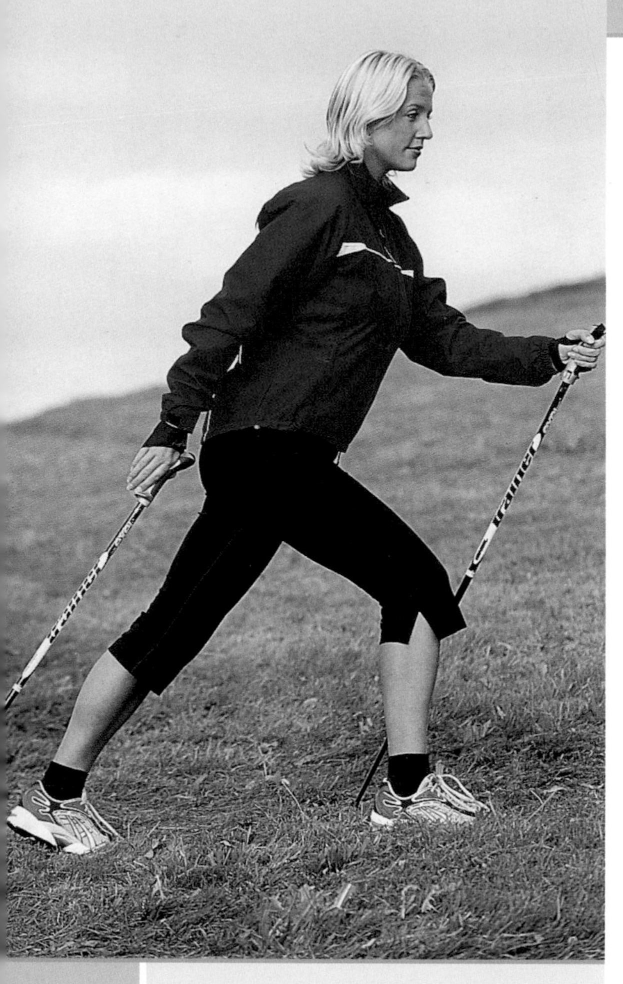

Your upper body should always lean slightly forward when walking uphill.

Uphill and downhill

Walking on a slope poses particular challenges to your fitness level as well as your technique. When descending the slope, a walker's joints are often unnecessarily strained. But if you know what you're doing, uphill and downhill walking can be a lot of fun and will bring a welcome change.

Walking uphill

When walking uphill you really have to give it your all if you want to maintain your speed and pace length. You can compensate for the higher exertion of your calves and knees by working your arms more. Try to distribute as much weight as possible to your walking poles. Lean your body as far forward as possible when walking uphill. But definitely make sure to unfurl your whole foot, despite the slope, and not just walk on the balls of your feet.

Walking downhill

To stop yourself from going too quickly when walking downhill, make your steps as small as possible. Always set the points of your poles behind your body and brake any acceleration by leaning backwards slightly. To take the load off your front leg, your weight should be distributed over the heel of whichever foot is positioned forward and the opposing walking pole – the more weight your pole is carrying, the better.

Besides this, it is also extremely important to keep your legs always slightly bent when walking downhill. This way your center of gravity stays as low as possible and the chances of slipping are reduced.

Training program for nordic walking

With the help of the training plan below, you can start Nordic walking even as a speed walking beginner, or switch over to Nordic walking after past experience. Experts will also find something for themselves here. In the beginning, it's best to walk more frequently and for shorter sessions. As soon as you start walking longer stretches you can reduce the frequency of your training.

Weeks 1 to 4

Begin your training with three to four sessions a week of 20 minutes each. Be sure to keep your movements clean and to use your walking poles in the proper manner. Your heart rate should be around 60 to 75 percent of the maximum pulse rate (see page 49). Try to increase your training time to 25 minutes in week four.

Weeks 5 to 8

In weeks 5 and 6 walk twice a week for 25 and 30 minutes, respectively, with a constant heart rate of 60 to 75 percent. In weeks 7 and 8 you should then be able to accomplish 30-minute training sessions 4 times a week.

Weeks 9 to 12

It should be no problem for you to walk 30 to 45 minutes at a time. Your pulse rate ought to be in the upper range of what you have so far achieved (75 to 80 percent of your maximum pulse), without running out of breath straight away. Only three training sessions per week will be sufficient at this training load. Continually challenge yourself. Beginning with the tenth week you can attempt to walk 60 minutes at a time without stopping. Your condition will be so good at this point that you can challenge yourself to walking on a gradual mountain slope.

INFO

TRAINING PROGRAM NORDIC WALKING

Weeks	**1–4**	**5–8**	**9–12**
Optimal heart rare (% of max. pulse)	60–75 %	60–75 %	75–80 %
Training time per session (in minutes)	20–25	25–30	30–45 +
Sessions per week	3–4	4	3

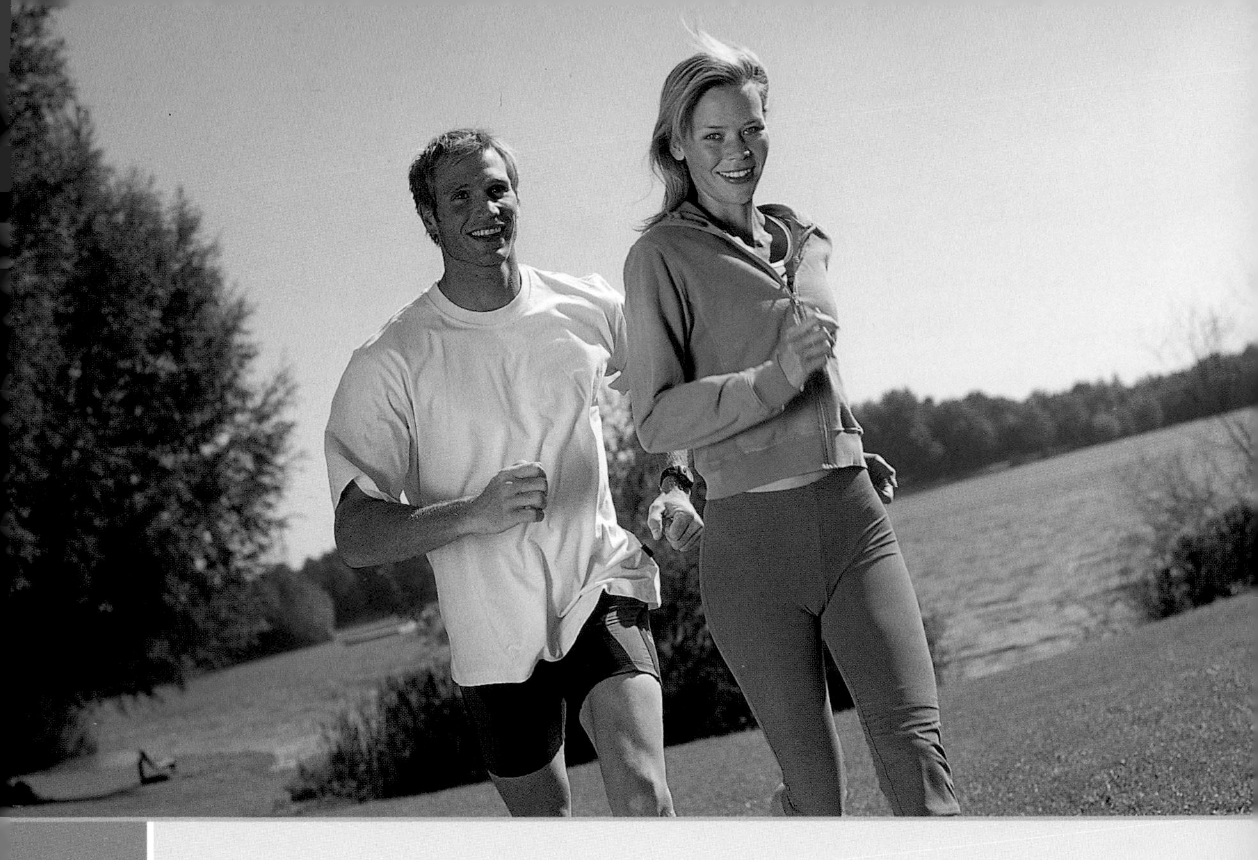

Light running

If runners and speed walkers did not use to have a lot in common, the situation today has changed somewhat. Speed walking is no longer considered a substitute sport for those who aren't capable of running.

And that's just fine! Speed walking and running can be combined in a way to form a light running program that may offer a welcome change to your daily training and pose new challenges.

Instead of exerting yourself to the point of injury, with light running you can dose out the exertion in such a way that your body will still be able to recuperate between training sessions. As with power walking interval training (see page 75), when training for light running, faster running phases alternate with slower speed walking phases. For this reason light running is ideal for beginners and reinitiates alike.

Power with pauses

Pulse rate can increase dramatically for jogging beginners because of the high speed. Inexperienced joggers will not only run out of breath this way, but they also over-exert their cardiovascular systems and burn less fat. After training they will feel exhausted and be in a bad mood. This isn't exactly the best motivation for repeating such training. With light jogging, however, and the stretching exercises between training sessions, you are ensuring that your pulse declines again or never shoots up in the first place. This way you will be training almost automatically within your optimal pulse rate.

Stretching between sessions

The loosening and relaxation of your muscles also play an important role when training for light jogging – and not only after your training session but between sessions as well. These periods of relaxation, as well as the medium pace at which you train, aid you in making it through each training session with ease, not least because your breathing can re-regulate itself and stretch your muscles when you relax, which contributes to additional relaxation.
You can find the best stretching exercises starting on page 34.

Training goals

Light running is a moderate endurance training for your fitness and your figure – ideal for anyone who wants to lose a few pounds or just do more for their heart and circulation. Beyond this, it helps to break down stress hormones in your body – and not just for the short term either. If you run regularly, you are better equipped to maintain peace and quiet, even in a hectic schedule. But this training program is also ideal for anyone who wants to switch over from speed walking to running, or who would like to train in both disciplines. The reason is that because of the constant alternation between walking and trotting, your body will slowly adapt to the higher strain and will be able to handle higher speeds over longer routes as well.

TIP

REGULATING YOUR PULSE

If your heart rate goes too high, simply switch over from running to speed walking or incorporate an extra stretching break into your training session.

Run and take off

With light running you combine the techniques of speed walking and jogging. You have already read (page 23) about which movements are best. With running it is also a matter of the optimal posture as well as the correct leg and arm motion. Unlike with walking, when you run, each foot is in the air for a short time with each step. There is no ground contact between pushing off and returning to the ground. Always make sure when running that, above all, you're moving forward! So, don't lift your feet too far from the ground. The higher you "fly", the farther you will fall when you come down. And that costs energy and puts strain on your joints. Finally, three times your body weight must be caught in when running.

Step by step

Your pace length is correct when your foot, when returning to the ground, comes exactly beneath your body's center of gravity. It's better to take several small steps ("trotting") than a few big ones. If you step too far from your center of gravity you will be braking your forward motion with every step you take. Another thing to practice is the positioning of your foot when meeting the ground after the short airborne phase. There is no universal technique but rather three various methods: walking with the middle of your foot, with the heel, and with the ball of your foot. Each technique has its own advantages and disadvantages.

Walking with the middle of your foot

This technique is recommended most of all for beginners and those with weight problems, as it helps to evenly distribute body weight. You land on the middle of your foot's outer edge, continuing with your heel down until you're standing on your entire foot. You then roll your foot forward to push off once more with the ball of your big toe. This technique is ideal on an open training ground.

Walking with your heels

When walking with your heels, first land with the outer edge of your heel to the ground and turn your foot inward as it declines until your sole is entirely on the ground. This technique is recommended when walking downhill or when you are attempting longer stretches. If you sense pain in your heels, ankles, knees, or spine you should switch to another technique.

Running on the ball of your foot

With this variant you first step with the ball of your foot on the ground. Only

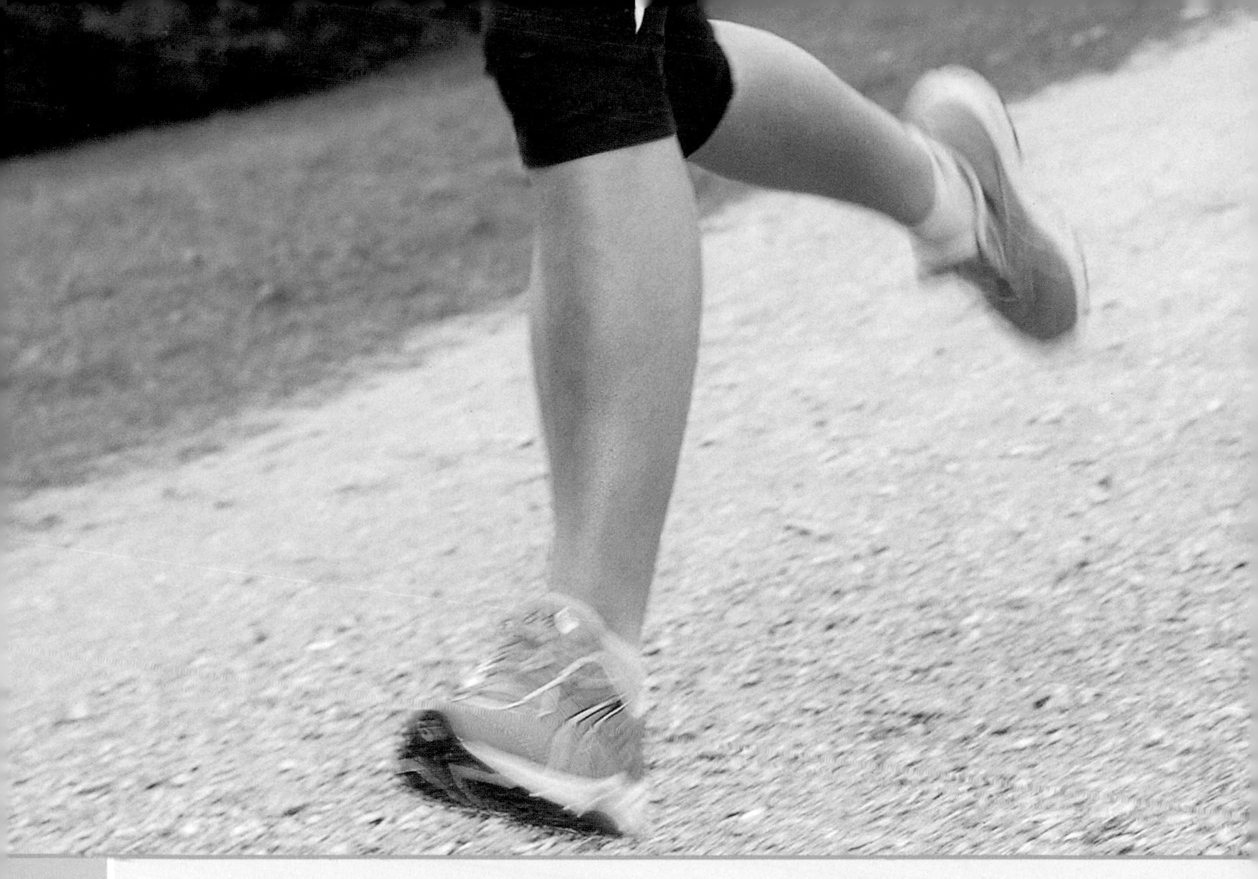

In a short airborne phase, both feet leave the ground for a moment when running.

then do you shortly place the middle of your foot and your heel on the ground to directly roll back once more to the ball of your foot. This variant is ideal for when you're walking uphill and is favored by sprinters. For light running without any need for high speed, you are better off choosing one of the other two techniques. You should also change your running style if you start noticing pains to your Achilles tendon or your calves.

Upper body and arms

As is the case with speed walking, you should keep your upper body straight when running as well. Keep your shoulders loose and drawn down slightly so that your back remains straight. Look a few yards ahead so that your neck and shoulder area does not cramp up and also to be able to dodge any obstacles in time. Your arms should be at about a 90-degree angle and should swing along loosely. Do not clench your hands into fists but keep them slightly open.

Training program for light running

Even just three 30- to 45-minute training sessions per week are enough to get the optimal use out of this light running training. The following program is suited to both beginners and advanced athletes.

Weeks 1 to 8

Run and walk for a total of 30 minutes per training session in the first eight days of the program. Including stretching, each should turn out to be about 45 minutes.

Run two to three times a week in weeks 1 to 4, then three to four times a week beginning with week 5.

Heart rate should be 60 to 75 percent during the entire training phase (see chart page 49).

Here's how:

- Warm up by speed walking for about 5 minutes.
- Fall into a light trot and run in this manner for 2 minutes.
- Reduce your speed once again and speed walk for one minute.
- Now it's stretching time (see page 34). Breathe deeply and calmly when stretching: stretch chest, neck, and back.
- Speed walk again for 1 minute.
- Increase your speed and run for 2 minutes.
- Speed walk for 1 minute.
- Run for 3 minutes.
- Speed walk for 1 minute.
- Run for 3 minutes.
- Speed walk for 1 minute at a medium pace, raising your arms above your body and breathing deep into your body while doing so. Lower your arms and breathe out slowly. Breathe normally again and raise and lower your arms.
- Run for 4 minutes.
- Speed walk for 1 minute.
- Run for 2 minutes.
- Speed walk for 4 minutes to a stop.
- Stretch well one more time: calves, upper thigh, and hips.

INFO

TRAINING PROGRAM LIGHT RUNNING

Weeks	1–4	5–8	9–12
Optimal heart rate (% of max. pulse)	60–75 %	60–75 %	75 %
Training time per session incl. stretching (in minutes)	45	45	60
Sessions per week	2–3	3–4	3–5

Weeks 9 to 12

Beginning with the ninth week, try to walk fast enough for your pulse rate to remain at 75 percent of your maximum heart rate throughout the whole training session (see chart page 49). Also increase the length and frequency of your training sessions one more time. Each week you should train between three and five times. Including stretching, each session should then come to 60 minutes. So, you're running and speed walking 15 minutes longer each time.

Here's how:

- Warm up by first speed walking for about 5 minutes.
- 2 minutes of running.
- 1 minute of speed walking.
- 3 minutes of running.
- 1 minute of speed walking.
- Now it's stretching time (see page 34 and following):
- Chest
- Nec
- Back
- 1 minutes of speed walking.
- 2 minutes of running.
- 1 minute of speed walking.
- 3 minutes of running.
- 1 minute of speed walking.
- 4 minutes of running.
- 1 minute of speed walking.
- 5 minutes of running.
- Speed walk for 1 minute at a medium pace, raising your arms above your body and breathing deep into your body while doing so. Lower your arms and breathe out slowly. Breathe normally again and raise and lower your arms.
- Run for 5 minutes.
- Speed walk for 1 minute.
- Run for 4 minutes.
- Speed walk for 4 minutes to a stop.
- Stretch well one more time: calves, upper thigh, and hips.

TIP

MEASURING YOUR TIME

To switch over from speed walking to running and vice-versa, it's best to train with a pulse watch that also displays the time.

Week 13 and following

Try to maintain the condition you have achieved after the twelfth week. Spend at least one hour three times a week training or replace a normal hour of speed walking with light running every now and again.

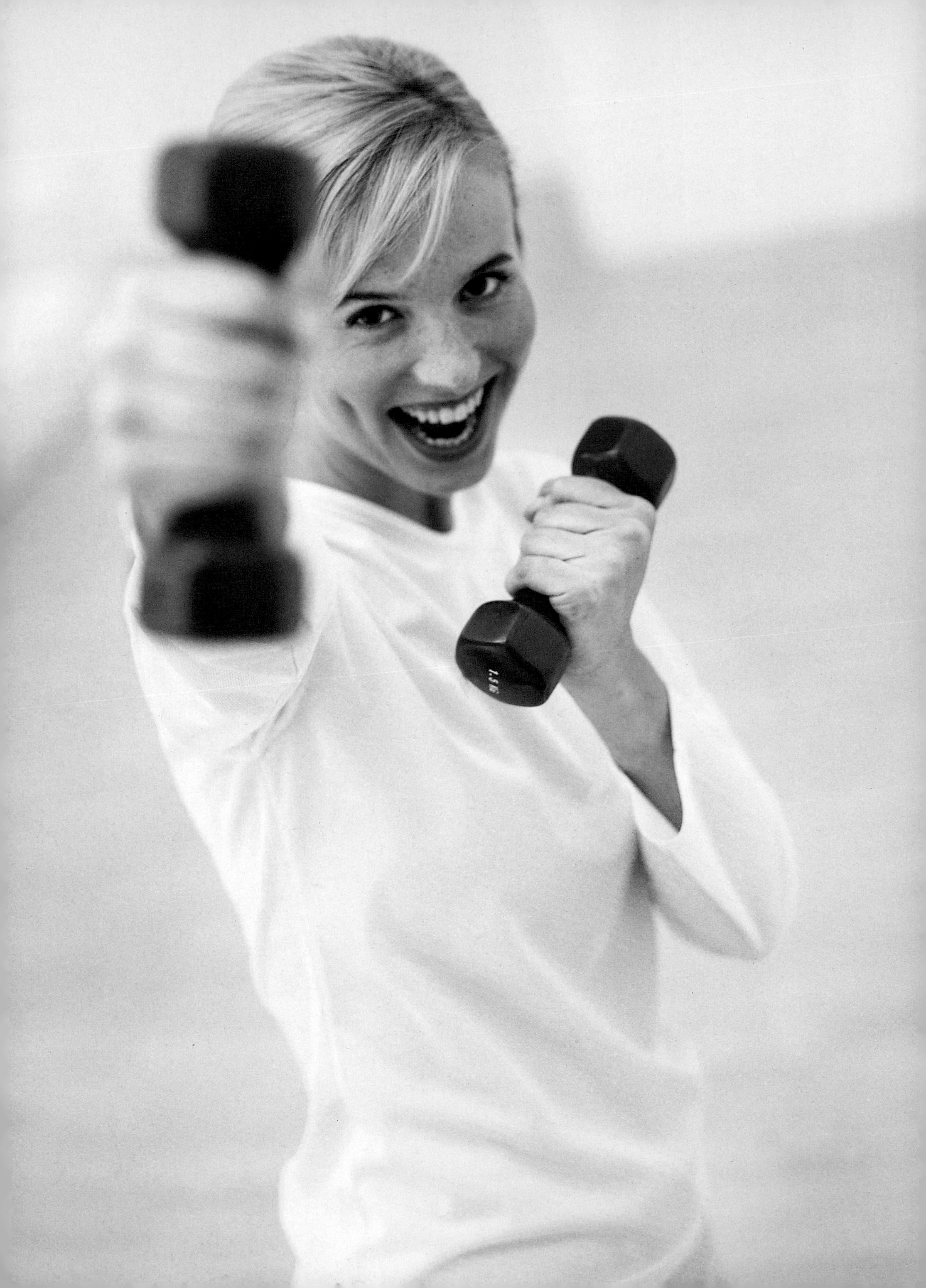

Walking specials

In this chapter you will find three walking programs that are specially adapted to meet various needs. With shape walking, the pounds will melt away and the accompanying workout will give you more muscle. Wellness walking is a mixture of meditative running and Asia wellness – ideal for tuning out. The final program is designed for pregnant women and for mothers with newborns who want to adapt speed walking to their present situation.

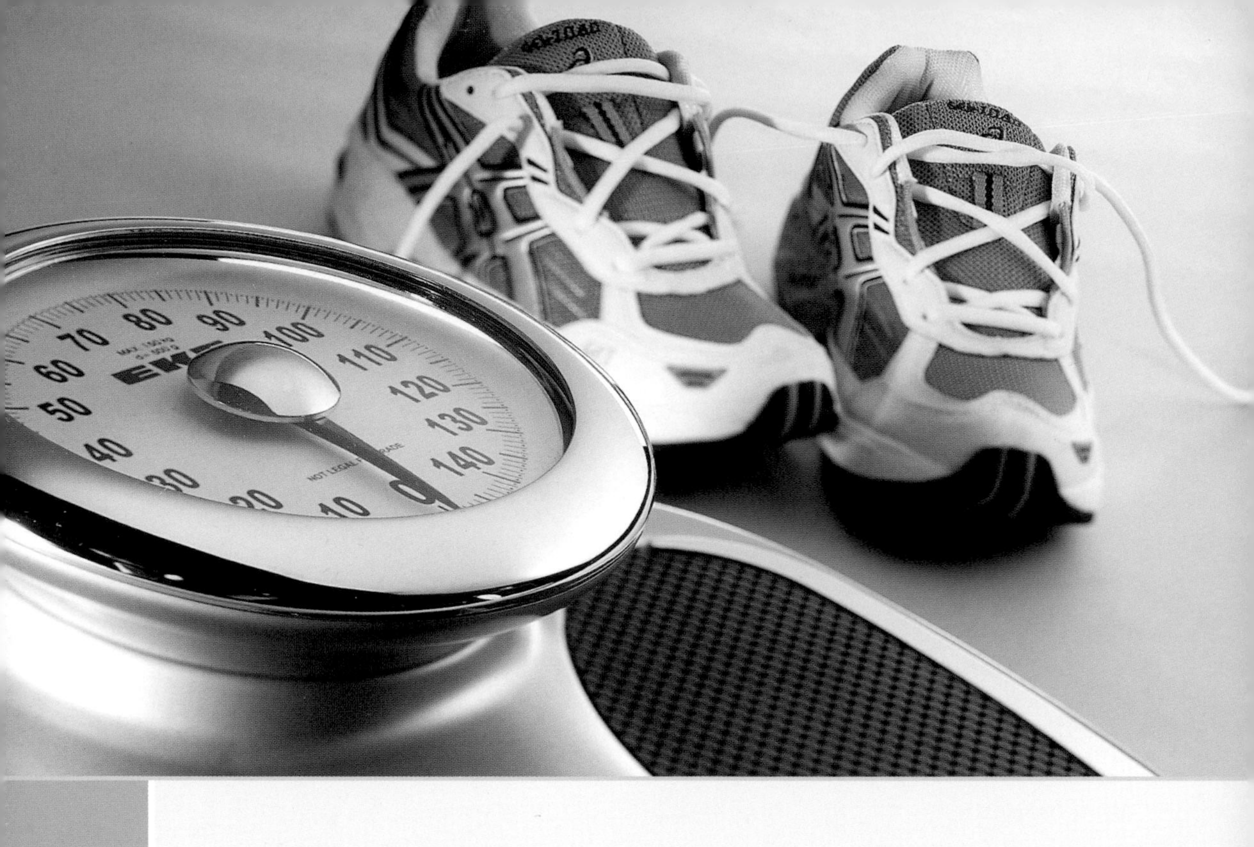

Shape walking

The ultimate goal of shape walking is to improve your figure. Naturally, this type of training, like every form of exercise, has a positive effect on your health and well-being. But the combination of endurance training and power exercise is simply unbeatable if you want to lose weight and tighten up your figure while you're at it. So you can forget all those miracle diets and hunger cures and start shape walking. If you exercise enough, tap into those fat reserves, and build new muscles the pounds will melt away for the long term. True, it might happen somewhat more slowly than with a crash diet. But as compensation you don't have to worry about the much-feared yo-yo effect. Of course, a balanced diet is also important. But as soon as you start training on a regular basis, your body will send you signals regarding its own needs. And what it usually needs are fruit, vegetables, and other "lightweight" foods.

Losing weight for good

Endurance training is the ticket to losing weight. You burn the most energy this way. And the only way to lose weight over the long term is for your body to burn more energy, calories, than it consumes. Not only this but through regular endurance training your body will learn to draw energy not only from the easily accessible carbohydrate reserves but to directly tap into those bothersome fat deposits.
The second secret of long-term weight loss is power training. The more muscles you have, the more energy you will burn. Finally, fat can only be burned by your muscles. And this doesn't only happen when you exercise! Because your energy-consuming basal metabolic rate increases, your body will be burning more calories even when you don't move. Every gram of muscle mass is, for this reason, an important step in the direction of your dream figure.

Shaping your figure

Even if you're generally satisfied with your weight level but would like to tighten those curves a little, then shape walking is the ideal program for you. While you stay fit, flexible, and productive through speed walking, the accompanying workout will stabilize your muscle mass and thus tighten your figure.

Training elements

Shape walking isn't just a matter of burning as many fat reserves as possible through endurance training. At the same time, you should be building new muscle mass. Muscles don't just shape your body, they burn surplus energy as well. This is why you should add a complete all-round workout to every training session. It will help you train important muscles. How often you train depends on which goal you want to achieve. If you want to lose a lot of weight, then you should shape walk five times a week and complete a total workout three times a week. If you only want to tighten up your figure, it's sufficient to shape walk three times a week, each time followed by the complete tally of exercises. With both variants it's important for you to let your body sufficiently recuperate from the new muscle strain. You should schedule at least one day between two workouts and only walk on this day or take a total break from your training. Sometimes less is more. In fact, if your body is not allowed to regenerate, then it won't have enough time to refuel its energy depots. Stamina doldrums and a lack of motivation are the result. After about six

weeks your body will have gotten used to the new demands made on it, and you can boost your training load to as much as five sessions per week.
Have you achieved your goal? Have you lost some pounds and put on some tighter curves? Do not make the mistake now of stopping your shape walking exercises. True, you don't have to train as often as previously, but two training sessions a week followed by the accompanying workout are still necessary to ensure long-term success.

Workout

Any concern about building too much muscle mass with power training is completely ungrounded. These light exercises very gently shape your body and simultaneously tighten your tissue. Also, they have been developed precisely for typical female "problem zones". Nonetheless, you should pay attention to your body's signals. If a certain exercise is too much for you or doesn't do you any good, simply skip it and continue with the next one. Try again later to see if it goes any better the second time round.
Power training isn't so much about brute weight lifting as it is about know-how. If you aren't interested in stronger muscle volume and are more intent on toning your muscles, it's best to train at low to medium intensity, but with many repetitions. You don't have to completely exhaust yourself. Only exert yourself until you have the feeling that you could go just a little bit further.
How often you need to exert certain muscles depends on your personal fitness level.

- Beginners should start with one to two exercises (rounds) with 15 repetitions each.

INFO

TRAINING PROGRAM SHAPE WALKING TO LOSE WEIGHT

Weeks	1–5	from 6
Optimal heart rate (% of max. pulse)	60–70 %	60–70 %
Walking training time per session (in minutes)	45	45–60
Walking sessions per week	5	5
Workout training time per session incl. stretching (in minutes)	45	45
Workout sessions per week	3	3–5

- Advanced athletes should increase to three to four exercises with 15 to 20 repetitions each.

Take a one-minute break between each exercise to let the muscles recuperate. Very important: When doing exercises in which the right and left sides of your body are trained separately, always do all of them first on one side before switching to the other side.

Speed walk before you power train

Although it would offer some diversion to break up a speed walking session with separate power exercises, for the fat burning process to really get underway, it's best to bring your speed walking session to completion before tacking a workout onto the end of your training. If the weather is nice you can work out in the outdoors. Because it's necessary with some exercises to lie down on the ground or a bench, though, this isn't to be recommended in every season. You can always begin your workout at home. In any case, you shouldn't take more than a few minute's break, to take off your jacket and shoes, for example, so that you won't have to repeat your warm-ups once again. If the break extends too long, you can always run in place for five minutes before working out or dance to your favorite music.

Really breathe!

One of the most common mistakes when training is the wrong breathing. We tend to hold our breath especially when we are really exerting ourselves. This is exactly the wrong thing to do. Always make sure to exhale when you exert yourself (that is, when you're flexing your muscles), and inhale again when relaxing your muscles. It often helps to exhale audibly through your mouth, as the sound will make you more conscious of your breathing.

INFO

TRAINING PROGRAM SHAPE WALKING TO A TIGHTER FIGURE

Weeks	1–5	from 6
Optimal heart rate (% of max. pulse)	60–70 %	60–70 %
Walking training time per session (in minutes)	30–45	30–45
Walking session per week	3	5
Workout training time per session incl. stretching (in minutes)	45	45
Workout sessions per week	3	3–5

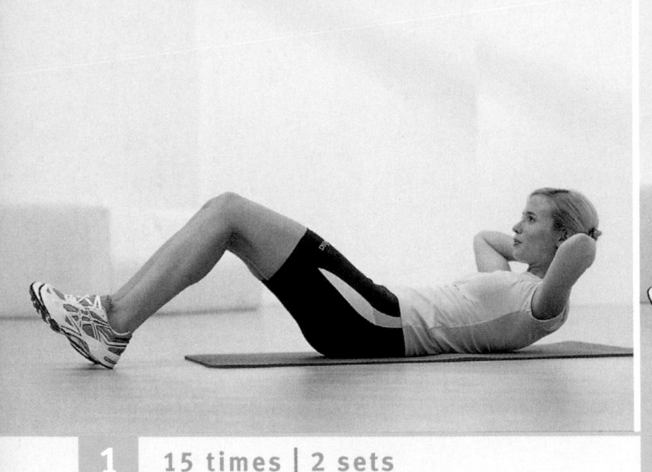

1 15 times | 2 sets

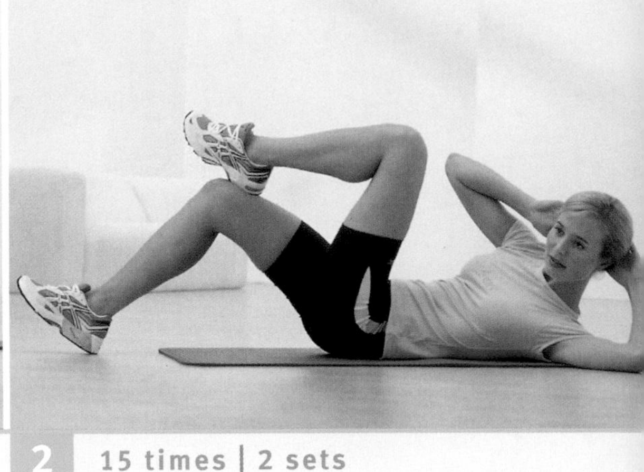

2 15 times | 2 sets

The best power exercises

With the following exercises you can train all the important muscles from head to toe.

Abdomen: Smooth muscle

- Lie down on your back, bend your legs and raise the tips of your toes from the ground. Support your neck in your hands with your elbows pointing outward. Flex the muscles in your stomach and push your lower back against the ground while doing so.
- Inhale. Slowly roll your upper body up from your lumbar vertebra (lower spine) to your chest vertebra (upper spine). Exhale while doing so. 1
- Hold the tension for a few seconds before slowly unrolling your upper body once more. Breathe in again while doing so.

Abdomen: Oblique muscle

- Return to the starting position for the smooth abdominal muscle training. Support your left foot against your right thigh. Suck in your stomach and push your lower back firmly against the ground as in the previous exercise. Inhale.
- Slowly push your right shoulder in the direction of your left knee. Your elbows should be pointing outward. Exhale. 2
- Hold the tension for a moment and return to the starting position. Inhale.
- Change sides after the appropriate number of sets.

Relaxing: After the above abdominal training, lie flat on your back and circle your belly button several times with your hand in a clockwise motion. This will help your muscles to relax and prevent cramps.

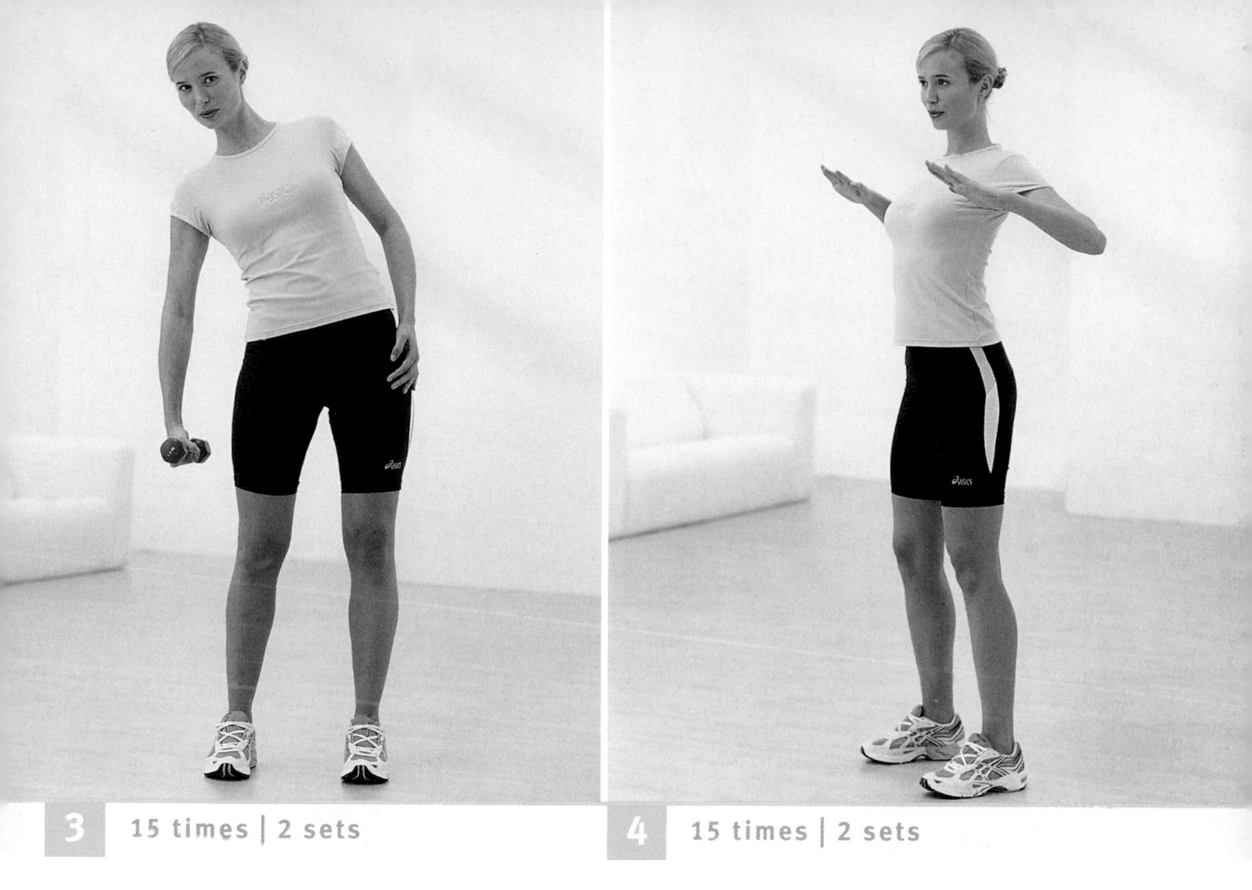

3 15 times | 2 sets

4 15 times | 2 sets

Waist

- Stand up straight with your legs open to shoulder width. Inhale.
- Bend your upper body to the right and run your left hand down along your leg as far as you can without tilting forward. Additionally, if you would like to intensify this exercise, you can try holding a two-pound dumbbell in your hand or a plastic bottle filled with water. Exhale while doing so. 3
- Slowly straighten your body and inhale again.
- After the appropriate number of sets, switch sides and repeat.

Important: When training your abdomen, you must always strengthen your back as well to prevent back pain.

Upper back

- Angle your arms at shoulder height to your sides. Your palms should face down, the tips of your fingers forward. Flex the muscles in your abdomen and rear. Inhale.
- Push your arms back and down two to four inches without tensing your shoulders as you do so. Exhale. 4
- Place your arms in a forward position once again, breathing in.

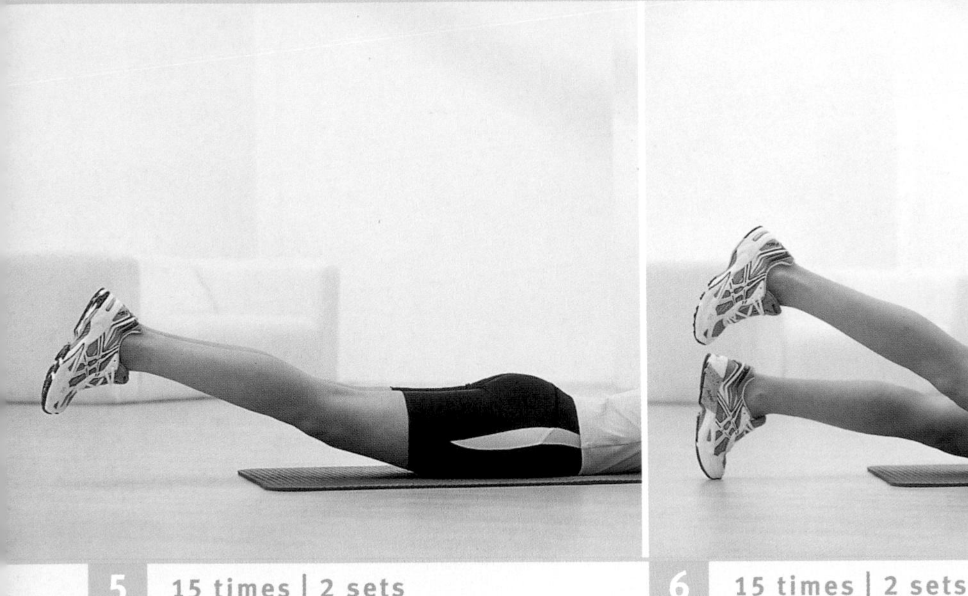

5 15 times | 2 sets

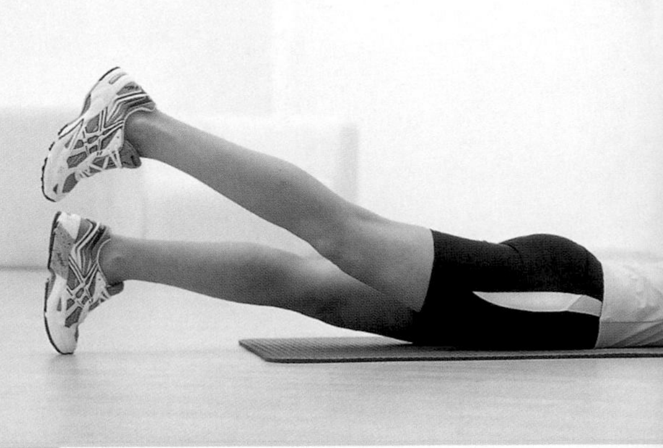

6 15 times | 2 sets

Lower back

- Lie down on your belly and support your forehead by leaning it on your crossed forearms. Place the tips of your toes on the ground, tense your rear, and push your belly against the ground. Inhale.
- Lift both feet a few inches from the ground and push them against each other. 5
- Hold the tension for five seconds and exhale while doing so. Lower your feet again without putting them down all the way and breathe in.

Buttocks

- Continue to lie on your belly. Place your toes on the ground, tense the muscles in your rear and abdomen, and breathe in.
- Slowly raise your right leg without bending it. Exhale while doing so. 6
- Lower your leg once again without the tips of your toes touching the ground. Inhale.
- After the appropriate number of sets, change sides.

Important: To prevent the development of saddleback while doing the exercises for your butt, you can place a rolled-up hand towel under your belly.

Quadraceps

- Stand with your legs open to shoulder width. Place your hands on your upper thighs. Inhale.
- Slowly push your rear down and back as if preparing to sit down in a chair. Your back should remain

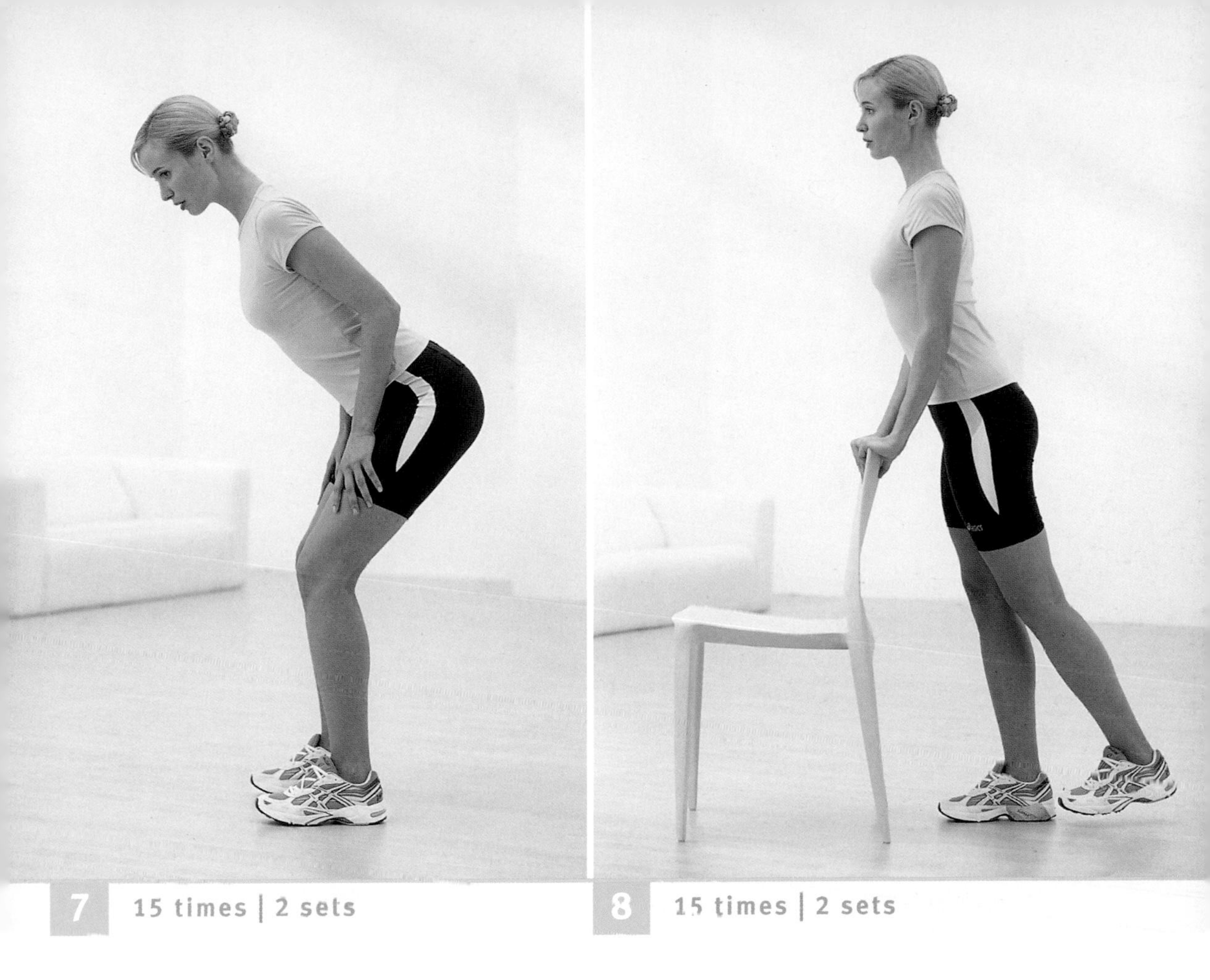
7 15 times | 2 sets

8 15 times | 2 sets

straight, your head and spine form a solid line. Exhale. 7

- Slowly return to the starting position and breathe in while doing so.

Important: Do not lower your rear too much. The angle between your calves and thighs must equal at least 90 degrees; otherwise your knees will be too greatly strained.

Hamstrings

- Stand up straight behind a chair and support yourself by gripping the chair back firmly with both hands. Shift your upper body forward slightly, back straight, to prevent saddle back. Inhale.
- Stretch your left leg straight back and lift it about eight inches. At the same time, point the tips of your toes outward and exhale. 8
- Lower your foot again without completely setting it down on the ground. Inhale while doing so.
- Switch sides after the appropriate number of sets.

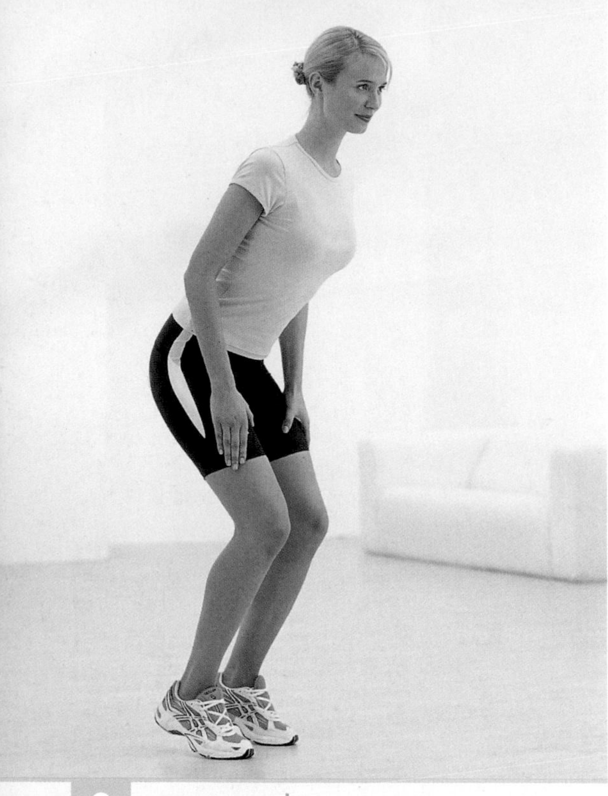

9 15 times | 2 sets

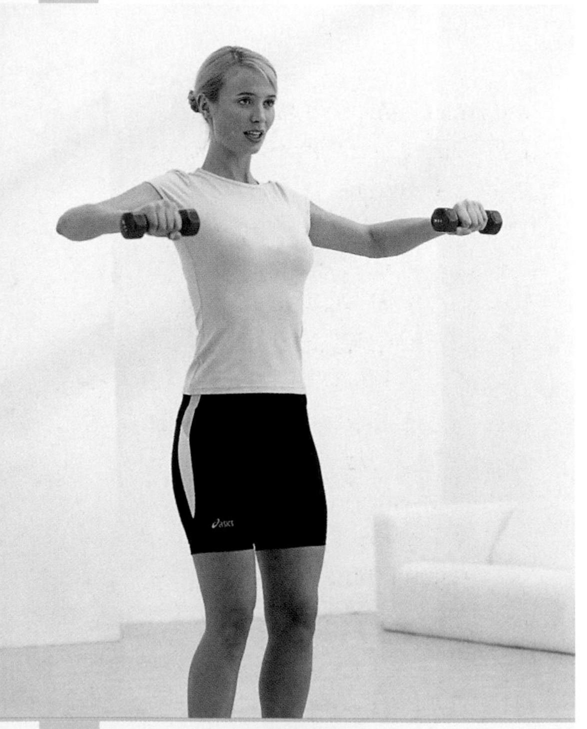

10 15 times | 2 sets

Calves

- Stand up straight with your legs open to shoulder width. Kneel down and rest your hands on your thighs. Inhale.
- Slowly lift your heels from the ground and count to five. Exhale while doing so. 9
- Slowly lower your heels once again without completely setting them down on the ground. Inhale.

Shoulders

- Stand up straight. Your legs should be open to shoulder width, your knees slightly bent. Hold a two-pound weight in each hand, or possibly a 40-ounce plastic bottle filled with water. Place your upper arms sideways to your body, your lower arms pointing forward at a right angle, palms outward. Breathe in.
- Gradually raise your bent arms up to shoulder height. Exhale while doing so. 10
- Slowly lower your arms once again without letting your upper arms touch your upper body. Breathe in.

Biceps

- Remain in the starting position and turn your lower arms in such a way that your palms are pointing upwards. Inhale.

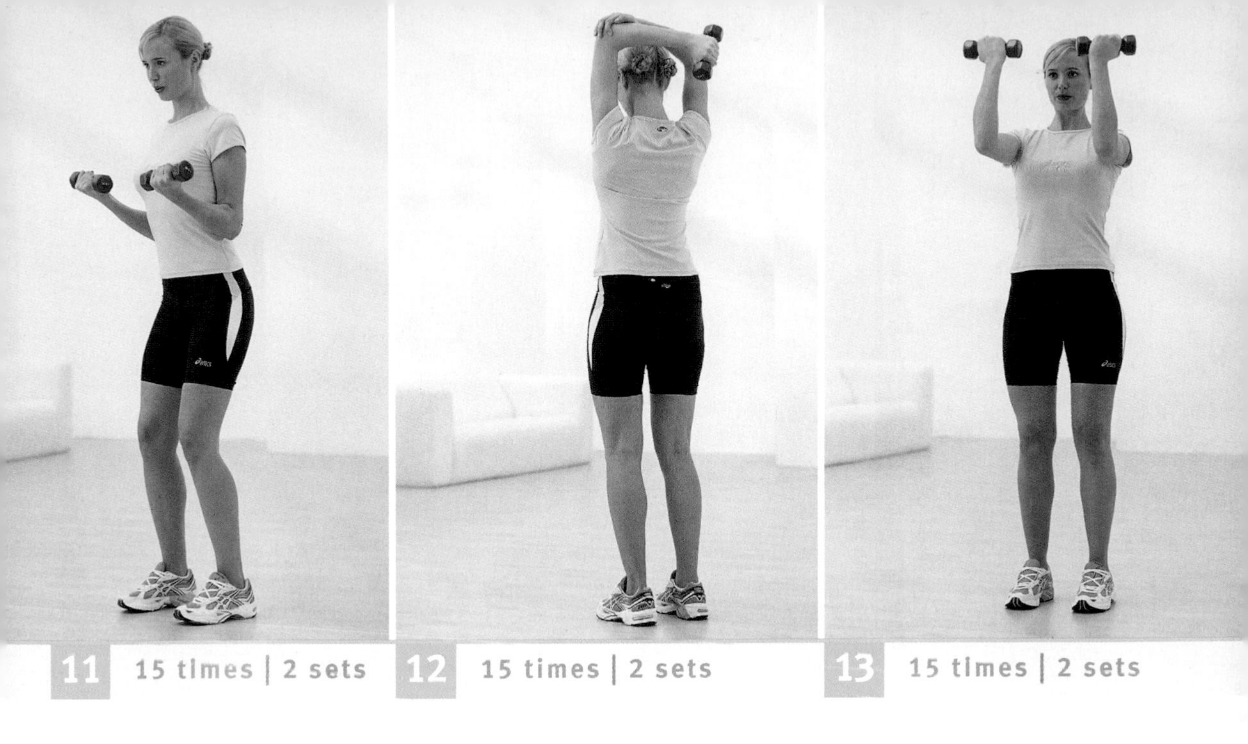

- Slowly raise your forearms until the angle between your upper and lower arms is just roughly 45 degrees. Exhale. 11
- Slowly lower your arms once again. Inhale.

Triceps

- Remain in this starting position. Your left hand holds a two-pound dumbbell. Angle your left arm and move it upwards behind your head. Your upper arm should be next to your head. Support your arm with your right hand on the elbow. Breathe in. 12
- Slowly extend your lower arm towards the ceiling without moving your upper arm. Do not completely extend your elbow while doing so. Exhale.
- Slowly lower your lower arm once again and breathe in while doing so.
- Switch sides after the appropriate number of sets.

Chest

- Remain standing and take both dumbbells in your hands one more time. This time, bend your arm in front of your body at a right angle and lift your upper arm to shoulder height. Place your lower arms together, thumbs pointing outward. Breathe in.
- Slowly move your arms about eight inches to the side without lowering your upper arms. Exhale. 13
- Slowly bring your arms back to the center and breathe in while doing so.

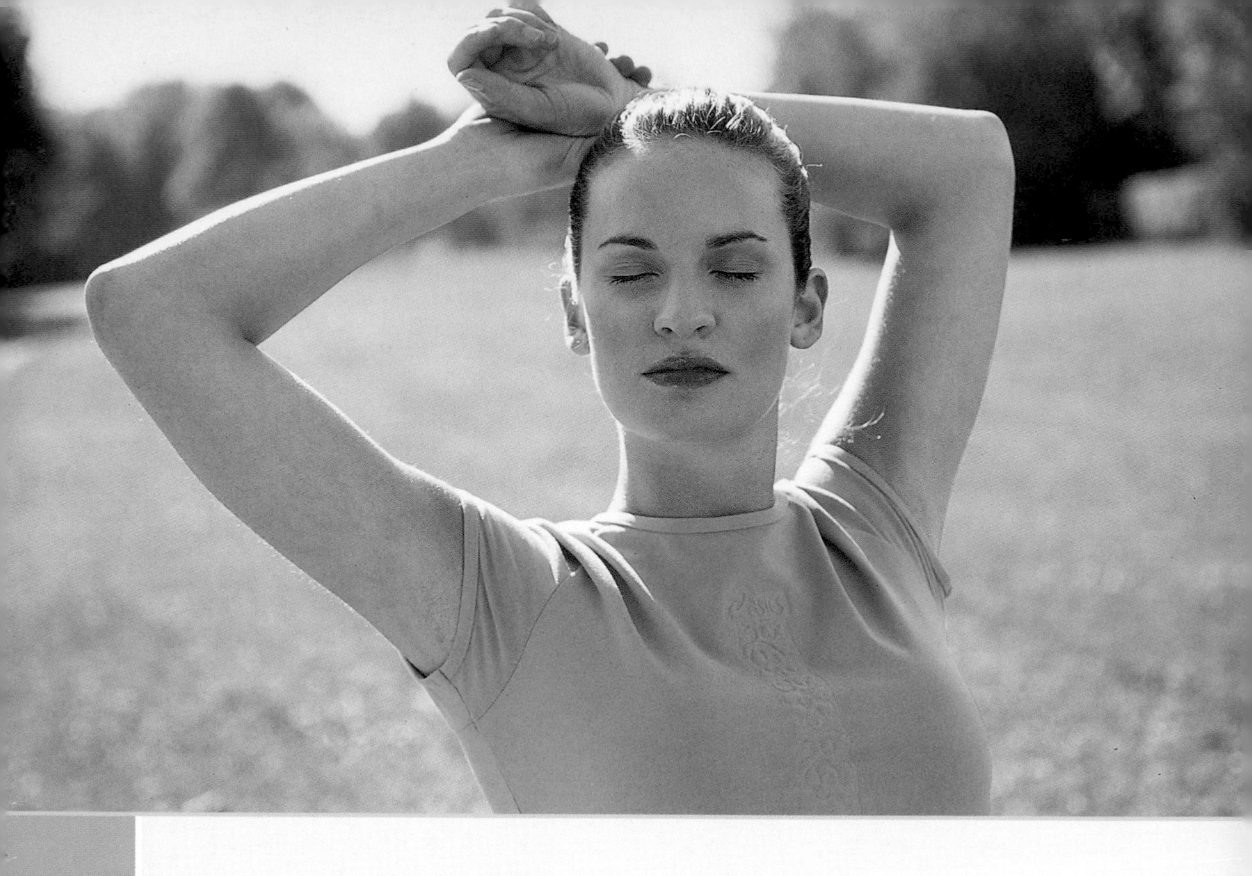

› Wellness walking

Exercise doesn't just keep you young and fit. If you are regularly active in sports, you will feel strong, self-empowered, and satisfied. You are more equipped to deal with daily encumbrances and suffer less from stress and exhaustion. In short: you simply feel more comfortable being you. If you find the wellness and enjoyment factor an important part of exercise, then the wellness walking program is tailor-made for you. It combines soft speed walking with walking meditations and empowering Asiatic relaxation methods such as Qigong and yoga. After such a training session, you will feel full of energy, as if reborn.
The movements involved in wellness walking are rhythmic and harmonious. They flow from one to the next and provide you with a sense of unity of body, mind, and soul.

Asia wellness

Besides the light exercise from speed walking, other exercises from Qigong and yoga can help you find inner peace and balance by breaking down stress and pressures in your body.
Qigong is a Chinese movement discipline dating back 5,000 years.
It helps to strengthen your Qi – the life energy that flows through certain channels, or meridians, in our bodies.
Using slow and fluid movements, concentration, and conscious breathing, inner blockages are dissolved, allowing this energy to flow freely once again.
Qigong helps against stress, exhaustion, back complaints, and circulatory disturbances.
Yoga is also much more than motion training. It influences our inner organs, breathing, heart rate, and blood pressure in a positive manner, reducing the stress hormones in your bloodstream.
The combination of speed walking, Qigong and yoga promises pure wellness.

Training program

There is no precise time frame for wellness walking. Beginners will initially have to walk longer than experienced walkers to achieve the relaxed, meditative condition at which the exercise aims. Pulse rate and speed also only play a merely secondary role. More important is keeping your breathing conscious and to maintain a conscious perception of your own body while rhythmically walking. Mentally focus on yourself and the life forces flowing into your body during these moments. You should plan between one and two hours for this training; in that time the desired effect should be achieved. The important thing is to perform the exercises from Qigong and yoga in a relaxed and conscious manner. It's better to leave some exercises out than to perform all of them at high speed. Otherwise, the desired easing of tension is quickly lost. There is, however, no upper limit. You can repeat each single exercise for as long as it does you good and gives you peace of mind.

TIP

EXPERIENCING NATURE

Wellness walking is particularly fun if you walk during sunrise or sunset and enjoy the early morning or late evening hours while doing so. Get a sense of how the sleepy world is waking anew or how a hectic day is ending in peace.

Soft walking: 1st lap

Look for peaceful surroundings without a lot of noise, crowds, or motor traffic. Concentrate on the program. Collect yourself, then breathe deeply.

- Relax your shoulders and mobilize your feet and your back (see page 31). Aim for soft, fluent, and harmonious movements, even during the relaxation exercises.
- Start off walking slowly. Your posture should be straight and comfortable, your body relaxed. Your mind should be still; concentrate only on your own walking. Increase your speed to a level you find comfortable.
- Sense how the air is flowing into your body, collecting there to flow onward into all the parts of your body. You mobilize your life force by breathing out: You open yourself up and clean your insides. Your breaths grow deeper and deeper.
- You can dissolve any tension with your breath. Guide it to those tense spots. Breathe "into your arm" or "into your belly". Feel how energy blockages dissolve and open the pathways for new energy to flow.
- Concentrate on the rhythmic movements of your walking. Feel how a wholesome fullness is spreading through your limbs. The fullness flows into your feet. Sense the ground beneath them! New power is flowing into you.
- Slowly become one with your surroundings. Open up your senses on all sides. With each breath you take the world around you is flowing, alive, into you. You feel like a small part of a wonderful, universal whole. Security and relaxation are expanding inside you. You feel like a drop of water in the river of life. Savor this moment of joy.
- Now interrupt your wellness walking for some Qigong exercises.

INFO

TRAINING PROGRAM WELLNESS WALKING

Walking training time 1	20–40 minutes
Qigong	10–20 minutes
Walking training time	20–40 minutes
Yoga	10–20 minutes
Optimal heart rate walking	60–75 % of max. pulse
Sessions per week	3–5

Qigong

Starting position

- Stand firm and still with your legs slightly open but not completely extended. Lean your pelvis forward somewhat. Your arms should hang down at your sides.
- Now very lightly raise your arms as if a pillow were stuffed beneath each shoulder. Turn your slightly arched hands in such a way that the tips of your fingers are facing each other as if invisibly connected. 1
- Stretch your head directly upwards as if it were secured to the sky by way of an invisible cord. Breathe deeply and with concentration for one minute. Then begin the exercise.

Reaching inner peace

- Remain in the starting position. Raise your hands up to your pelvis as if holding a bowl. The tips of your fingers should be pointing towards each other.
- As you breathe in, guide your arms upward in front of your body without raising your shoulders. 2
- Turn your palms downward at eye height and push your hands slowly down again. Exhale slowly and deeply while doing so. 3
- Repeat the exercise at least four times in total.

1

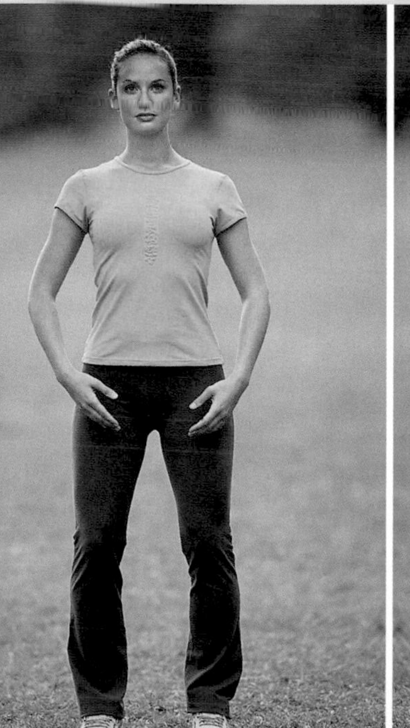

2 4 times

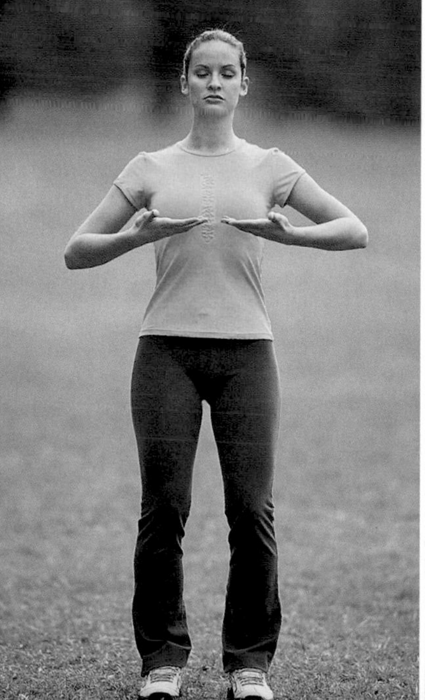

3 4 times

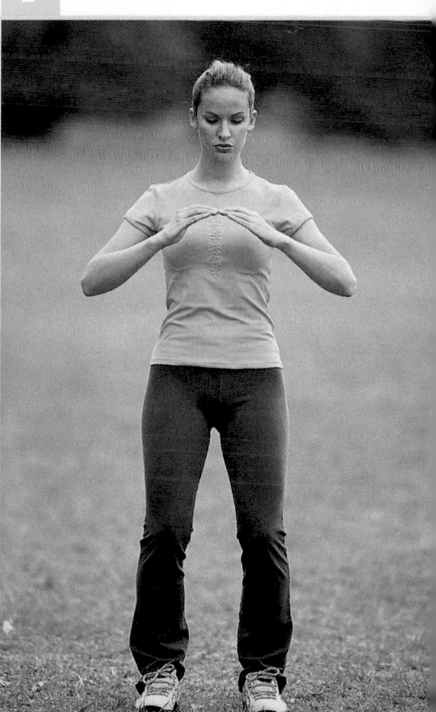

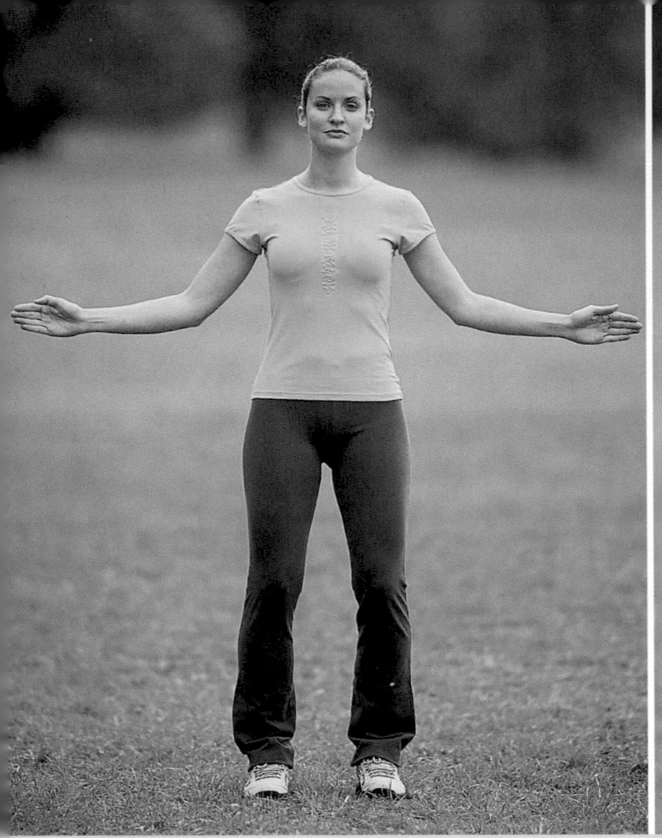

4 3 times

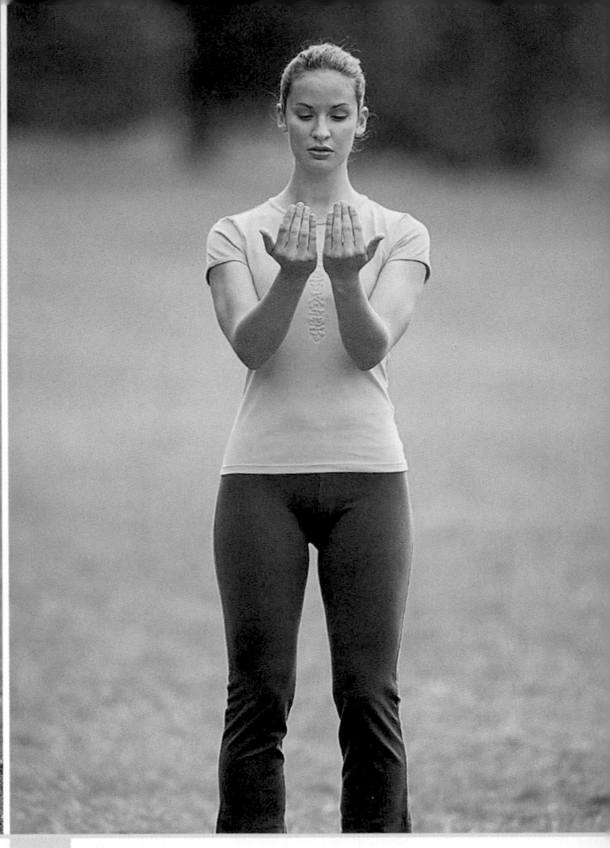

5 3 times

Clutching the sky

- Place your hands in the starting position once again. Then raise your arms sideways. When your arms form about a 30-degree angle to your body, turn your hands in a fluid motion so that the palms are now pointing straight ahead. 4
- Raise your arms higher until they are even with your head. Turn your hands once again so that the palms point down and your thumbs point out.
- Slowly lower your arms in front of your body again, as if they were carrying a bowl. 5
- Repeat the exercise three times.

Driving away the everyday

- Return to the starting position. Take an initial step forward with your left leg and place your weight on that leg. Simultaneously bend back your slightly angled arms.
- Put your arms forward, hands raised. Your palms should also point forward, as if they were pushing a burden away from themselves. Follow the line formed by your right leg while you do so. Do not turn outside of this axis and do not completely extend your arms. 6

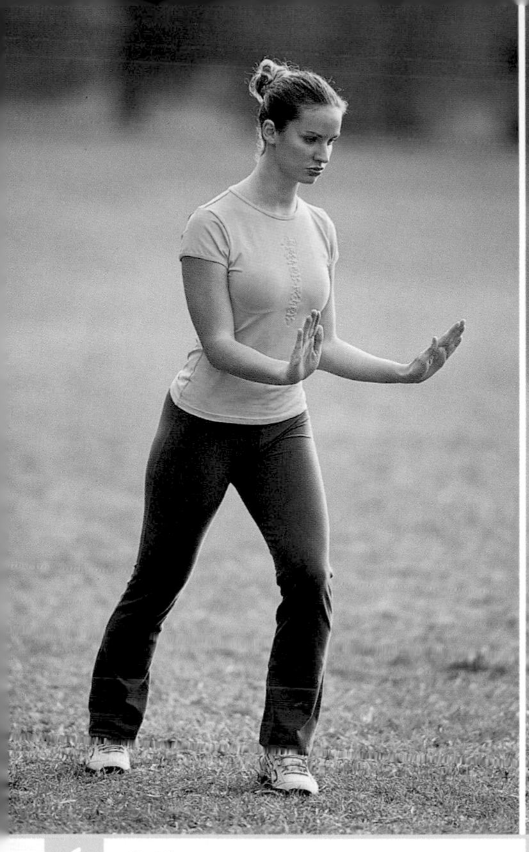

6 2 times

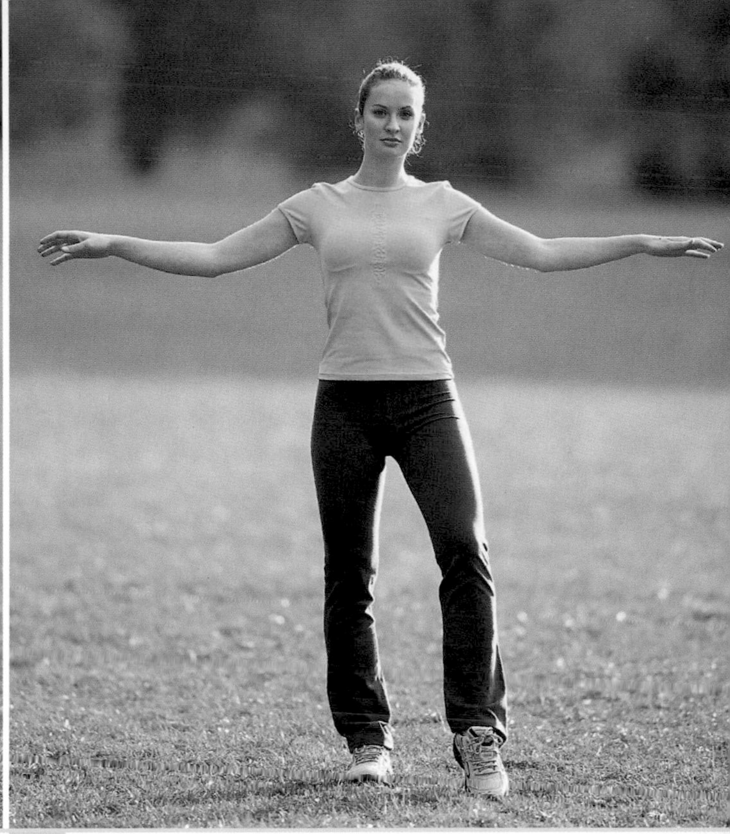

7 2 times

- Turn your palms inward so that they are facing you and bring your arms slowly back to your body again. Simultaneously bring your leg back again and return to the starting position.
- Change legs and perform the exercise on the other side.
- Repeat the exercise at least twice for each side.

Spreading your wings

- From the starting position, take an initial step forward with your left leg. Only step with the ball of your foot and place your weight on your right leg.
- Cross your hands once in front of your belly, then slowly spread out your arms up to roughly shoulder height, as if they were wings. Do not completely extend your elbow while doing so.
- "Swing" yourself in light, round motions through the air, without moving your upper body as you do so. 7 Consciously feel the sense of well-being that the exercise instills in you.
- Repeat the exercise at least twice for each side.

Qigong closure exercise

- Enclose the area around your kidneys four times with both hands flat.
- Bring your hands forward, keeping them tight to your body, and let them rest a moment just beneath your belly button. Breathe deeply.

Soft walking: 2nd lap

Start walking slowly. Increase your speed according to your need and speed walk as you did in the first lap (see page 106). Slowly reduce your speed at the end of the lap until you come to a complete stop.

8

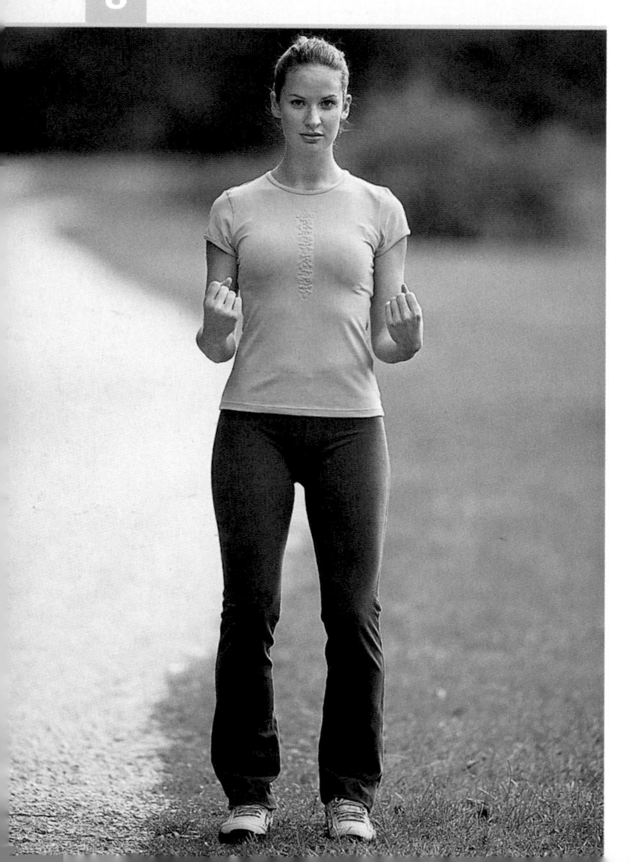

Take a firm, relaxed standing posture. The heaviness in your body will sink down into your feet, which connect to the earth like the roots of a tree. Energy flows from the ground over your feet and into your body. Now perform the following exercise.

The return

This exercise will ensure that you are relaxed, clear-headed, and tranquil for the rest of the day. Skip this part if you intend to go to sleep after the program.

- Close your hands into fists, tense your arms firmly, and swing them several times against your body. 8
- Now breathe deeply and audibly in and out several times. Relax all your muscles as you do so and look around with open eyes.

Yoga

Once you've returned home, you can add a relaxing yoga session onto the end of your wellness walking session. This will simultaneously function as a light stretching exercise.

Cat's Hump and Dog's Back

- Go down onto all fours. Hold your body up on your hands and knees. Your hands should be below your shoulders.

- Hang your head, pull your chin to your chest, and push your back upward to make a hump like a cat. Hold this position for roughly two minutes. 1
- Put your head into your neck, lower your back, and let it hang down (slightly saddle-backed). Freeze in this position for around two minutes.

The crocodile

- Lie down on your back. Bend your legs and lift up your feet. Your arms should lie beside your body on the ground.
- Let your bent knees sink to the left and turn your head to the right. Your shoulders should remain touching the ground while you do so. Hold this position for 30 seconds and breathe deeply and calmly in and out. 2
- Return to the starting position. Let your knees sink to the right while turning your head to the left. Repeat this exercise a minimum of three times through.

The seesaw

- Remain lying on your back and pull your knees up to your chest. Hug your knees with both arms and close your eyes. 3
- Swing softly to the left and right for as long as it feels comfortable.

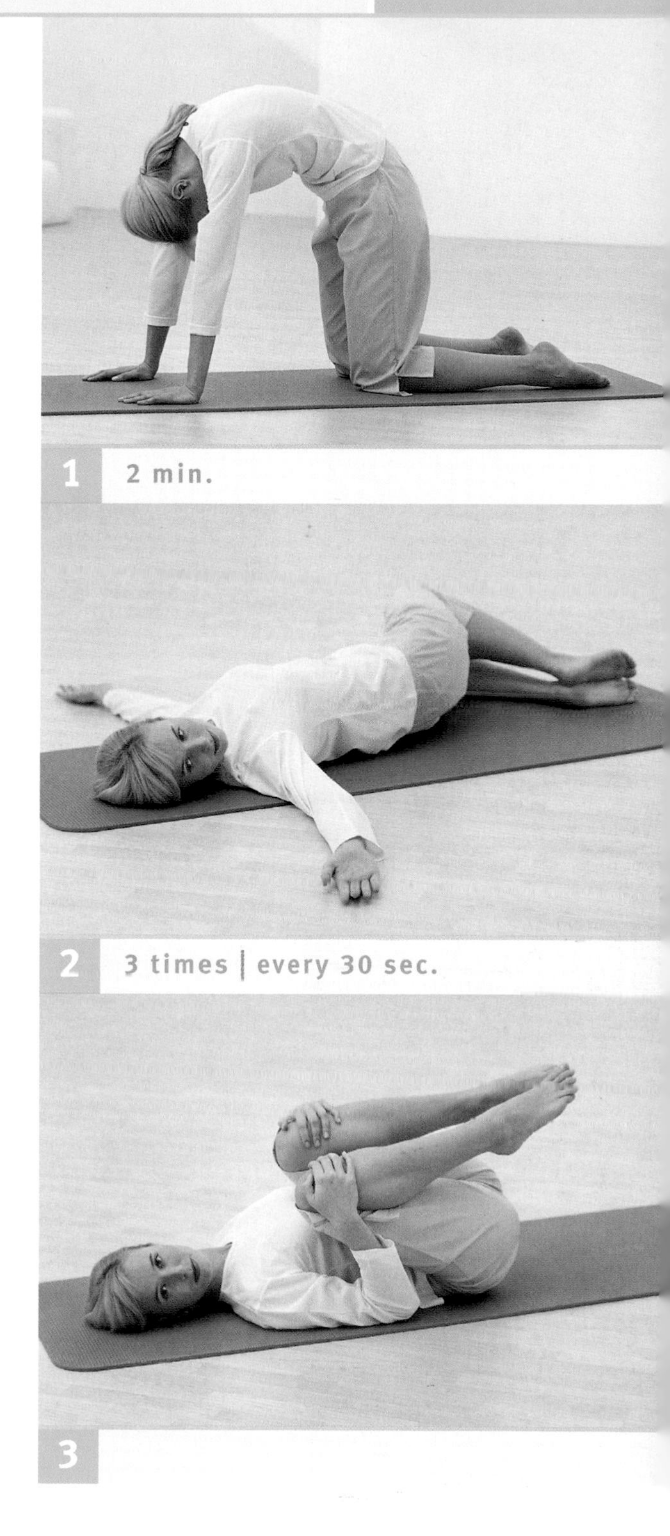

1 2 min.

2 3 times | every 30 sec.

3

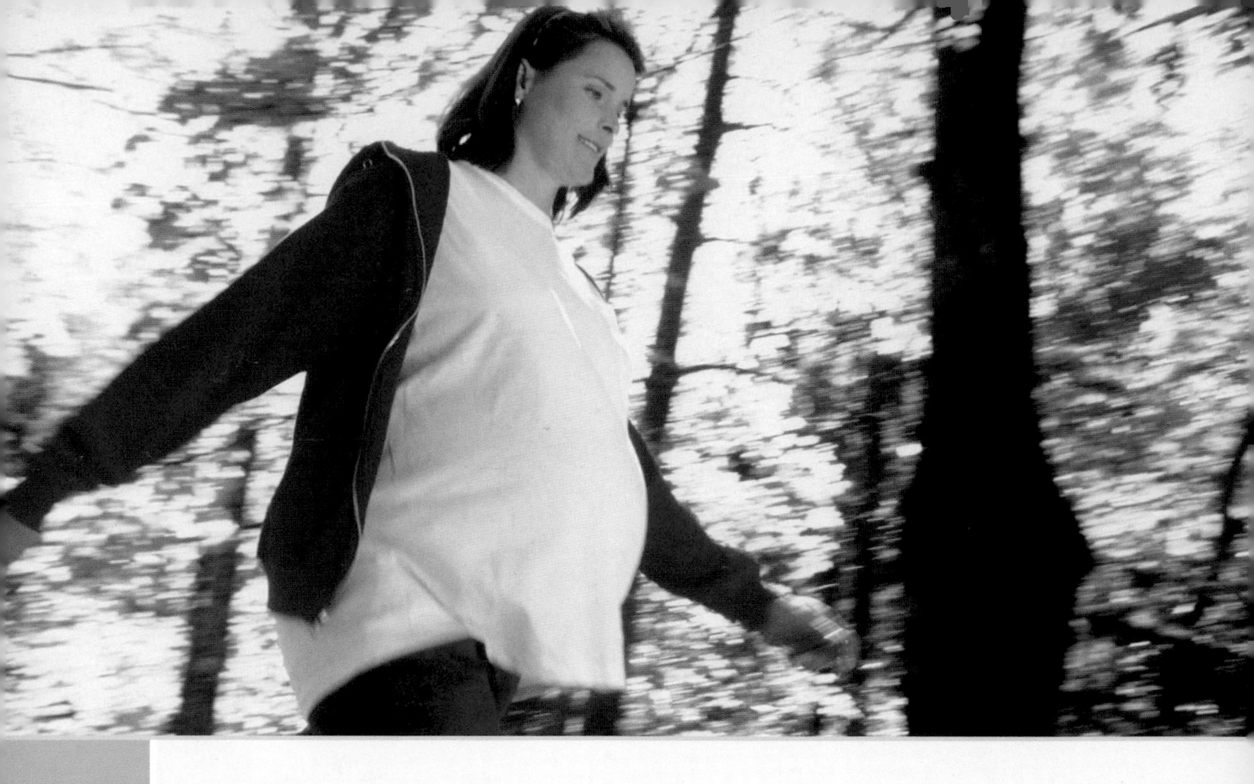

Walking with baby

Whether with a baby in your belly or in a stroller – there is (almost) no reason why mothers (and mothers-to-be) should avoid speed walking. As a soft sport, it is very well-suited for this period in your life and has a positive effect on the baby in your belly too.

Speed walking during pregnancy will help you stay fit and optimally prepare you for giving birth. The strains of pregnancy and birth can be handled better by an exercised body than by an untrained one. Also, the weight loss and re-adaptation that take place after birth usually go more quickly and with fewer complications for women who exercise. This kind of walking helps the mother reach her original fitness level quickly and easily.

The only important thing is that you do not over-exert yourself, neither during pregnancy nor after giving birth, and that you always train in the aerobic range for optimal oxygen intake. Consider that your sense of well-being is what matters, not some athletic achievement.

Walking pregnant

If your pregnancy is transpiring without any complications, you can continue walking without any problem at all. But make very sure that you walk at a moderate exertion level and in the aerobic range, with oxygen surplus. This means that you walk without high exertion and in such a way that you could carry on a conversation with someone.

Just think, your well-being should always be in the foreground, not athletic achievement.

If one of the following complications appears, you should speak with a gynecologist before you start walking:

- heart disorders
- infections
- pains in your belly or your chest
- previous, repeated miscarriages or premature deliveries
- grave problems during previous pregnancies
- premature labor
- hemorrhages
- premature dilation of the uterine orifice or shortened cervix
- meager growth of the fetus
- dizziness, headaches, or general feelings of unwellness
- an unusually high rate of water retention (edemata)

Target for speed walking during pregnancy

You can prevent typical pregnancy complaints such as back pain, varicose veins, stretch marks, or thrombosis by speed walking. This training improves your circulation on all levels and so leads to an optimal oxygen intake for both mother and child. Additionally, weight gain is usually less in the case of women who exercise regularly while pregnant than it is for those who do not. The birth is often easier as well.

And you're doing something good for your child when you walk. If you yourself feel fit and healthy, then you're giving your child the best possible chances for development. The child's sense organs are additionally stimulated by the soft swaying movements.

AVOID LYING ON YOUR BACK AFTER THE FIFTH MONTH!

IMPORTANT !

In very rare cases, the expanding womb can press against the vena cava, the superior hollow vein leading to the right atrium of the heart, thereby reducing blood flow to this organ. The baby will be supplied with too little oxygen. To prevent vena cava syndrome, you should lie on your left side during pregnancy.

Training program for pregnant women

You will find recommendations for training during pregnancy in the chart below.
Take special care to not over-exert yourself when training. If you become exhausted and run out of breath, or if you feel overheated, there is a danger of your child not getting sufficient oxygen and this can lead to other problems. Definitely plan for breaks and reduce the intensity of your training as soon as you begin to feel unwell. Train exclusively in the aerobic range. In this range, your heart rate should not exceed 75 percent of the maximum pulse rate (see chart, page 49). A rule of thumb: it's better to walk slowly over a longer stretch than to walk quickly for a short distance, and be sure to recuperate for at least one day between training sessions.

Warming up

Properly warming up and cooling down is especially important during pregnancy because blood flow is increased, fluids are retained, and the mother's heart must pump more. A good warm-up (five minutes) is not only good for your heart but for your muscles, tendons, and ligaments as well. These are subjected to increased loads during pregnancy due to the increase in body weight and hormonally-induced softening of tissues.

INFO

TRAINING PLAN FOR PREGNANT WOMEN*

	1st–4th month	5th–7th month	8th–10th month
Training heart rate** (% of max. pulse***)	B: 60–65 % A: 60–70 %	B: 60–70 % A: 60–75 %	B: 60–65 % A: 60–70 %
Walking on even terrain (briskly)	B: 10–20 min. A: 20–30 min.	B: 15–25 min. A: 30–45 min	B: 5–10 min. A: 10–20 min.
Cool down	5 min. energetically 5 min. stretch	5 min. energetically 5 min. stretch	5 min. stretch
Total duration	B: 25–35 min. A: 35–45 min.	B: 30–40 min. A: 45–60 min.	B: 15–20 min. A: 20–30 min.
Sessions per week	2	2–3	2

* Letters represent months of pregnancy – ** B = Beginners, A = Advanced
*** Maximum pulse rate defined as 220 minus age in years

Your muscles, tendons, and ligaments will have better circulation if you slowly warm them up before you start training, thus increasing their ability to cope with pressure (see page 31).

The appropriate workout

Just like the warming up phase before training, a well-planned cool-down belongs in every training session. You speed up the important process of regenerating those parts of the body that have been most strained.

It is a good idea to complement your speed walking training with some appropriate gymnastic exercises. Because of weight gain during pregnancy, which mostly concerns the belly, your muscles and spine are subjected to some major changes. Additional gymnastic exercises contribute to a strengthening of muscle mass and relief for the spine. Your body's load bearing capacity is increased this way and disorders such as back pain are prevented. Some suitable exercises:

- upper back (page 99),
- biceps (page 102),
- triceps (page 103) and
- waist (page 99).

Very Important: You should only train with weights for the triceps and waist exercises during the first third of your pregnancy! Perform these exercises as an addition to your speed walking session, preferably before warming up.

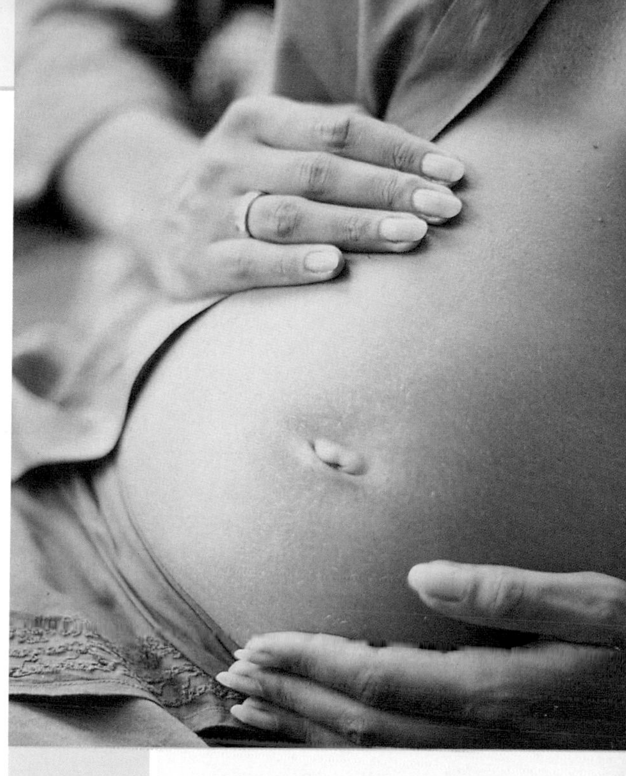

Neither before nor after birth is a baby an obstacle for speed walking.

As a supplement to your training, there are exercises meant to be performed standing and in the outdoors. You can complete additional gymnastic exercises at home and lying down. These can be learned at a birth preparation course.

During pregnancy, however, you should not train your smooth abdominal muscle, as this can lead to an enlargement of rectus diastase (the opening up of smooth abdominal muscle). Strengthening of oblique abdominal muscles during the first two-thirds of your pregnancy is completely safe and advisable.

Breathe deeply and evenly!

Only deep belly breathing, not just from your chest but your belly as well, can ensure sufficient oxygenation. This is the prerequisite for aerobic training. Make sure that you breathe out just as long, or even longer, than you breathe in. This way your lungs are able to completely empty themselves and you prevent side pains.

Drink enough fluids!

Sufficient hydration is especially important during pregnancy and is necessary for the replacement of amniotic fluid and increased blood content in your body. It's best to drink before you get thirsty. Water, sparkling fruit juice, or herbal tea are all ideally suited to compensating for fluid loss during speed walking and preventing dehydration during training.

Adjust your training

A woman's capacity for strain differs greatly in the three trimesters of pregnancy. The least complaints appear during the second trimester (the fourth to sixth months) so that you can carry on your training during this period without any problem.
During the first trimester (first to third months) it can be very difficult for many women to exert themselves physically due to nausea, vomiting, enervation, or dizziness. Pay good attention to such signals from your body and adjust your training to meet your body's needs. Walk slowly and set small distances as a goal for

TIP

DO YOU NEED A BABY BELT?

The "baby belt" supports your belly as it becomes larger and heavier. This can be quite pleasant when walking. You can also prevent lumbago and back pain this way. After delivery, a baby belt will support your physical reconditioning.

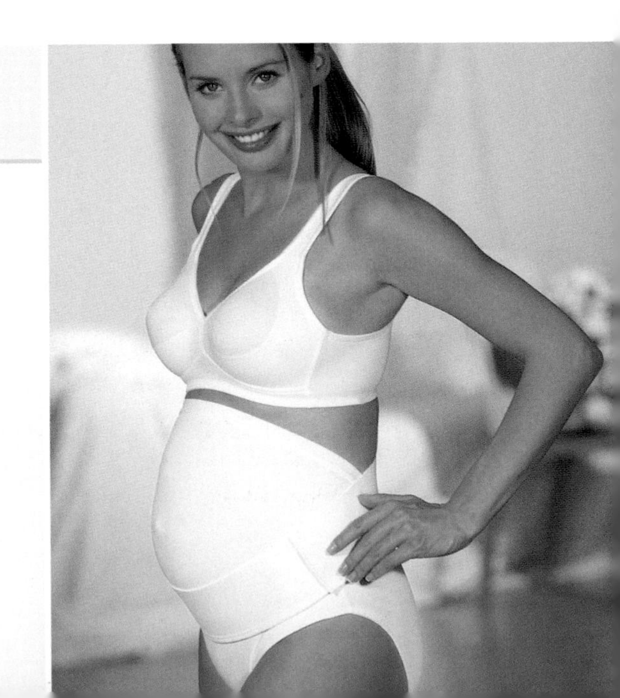

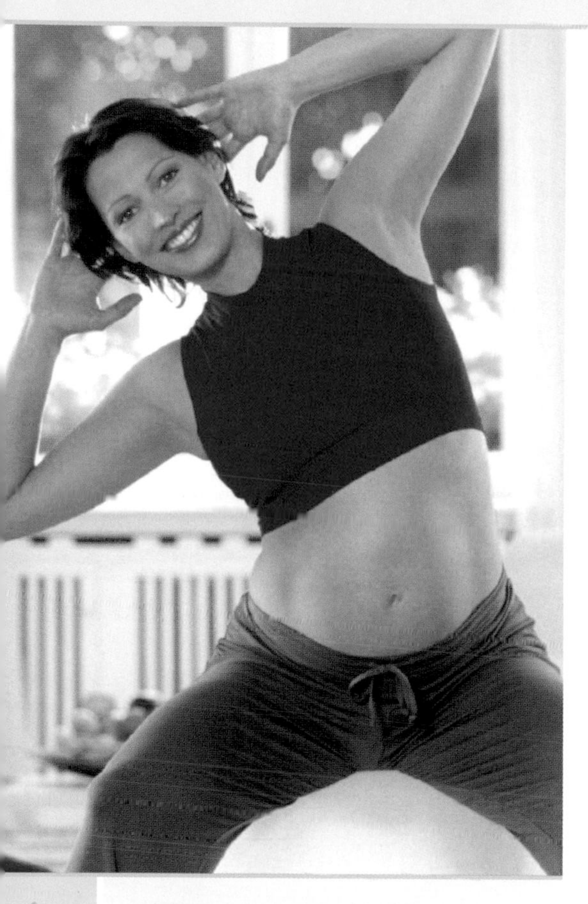

Light gymnastic exercise is also permissible when pregnant.

yourself. This way you have a good chance of actually decreasing such feelings of exhaustion and nausea by the soft movements in the open air. During the trimester (seventh to ninth months) you should also adapt your training to your ever-increasing belly. Then you can continue walking without any trouble right up to the day you give birth, as long as you feel well. It's advisable to supplement your training with relaxation exercises, especially in the last third of your pregnancy.

Post-natal walking

Pregnancy and birth make very high demands on a woman's body, so you should just allow your body to rest during the first eight weeks after you give birth. After a spontaneous delivery without any particular complications, however, you can start with a light speed walking training after only six weeks.
In the case of pregnancy or delivery complications such as gestosis (toxemia of pregnancy) or a caesarian section, you should certainly discuss your training plans with your gynecologist.

Post-natal walking targets

Walking training after delivery contributes to a recovery of your original figure and fitness level, to activating your circulatory system, and to tightening your tissue. Beyond this, it offers an outstanding possibility for relaxation and compensation for the everyday routine. You're doing something for yourself – and your baby, if you bring it along. Enjoy the peace and quiet and the exercise in the open air.

Training program for mothers

You can take up training after delivery once you feel somewhat fit again and your pelvis is stable. You will recognize this when you can hold your water and the base of your pelvis can be tensed when you sneeze. Fundamentally, what was important during pregnancy is important now as well (see page 113). Orient yourself for training by the following chart. Always pay attention to how you feel during training and do not over-exert yourself. Remember, now as always: it's not about athletic achievement.

Training and nursing

To be able to properly nurse your baby you have to consume enough calories from healthy foods and should not lose weight too quickly. In no case should you lose so much that you weigh less during the nursing phase than you did before pregnancy. When this happens, toxins will be set loose from stored body fat, which will be passed on to your child by way of your milk. If your baby is not growing as it should, this might be a sign that your training is too intensive and you are burning too many calories by speed walking.

INFO

TRAINING PROGRAM FOR MOTHERS*

	from the 6th week	3rd month	from the 4th month
Training heart rate** (% of max. pulse***)	B: 60 % A: 60 %	B: 60–65 % A: 60–70 %	B: 60–75 % A: 70–75 %
Walking on even terrain (briskly)	B: 5–10 min. A: 10–15 min.	B: 10–20 min. A: 20–30 min.	B: 15–30 min. A: 30–45 min.
Cool down	5 min. energetically 5 min. stretch	5 min. energetically 5 min. stretch	5 min. stretch
Total duration	B: 15–20 min. A: 20–25 min.	B: 25–35 min. A: 35–45 min.	B: 30–45 min. A: 45–60 min.
Sessions per week	1	2	2–3

* Figures in weeks or months after delivery – ** B = Beginners, A = Advanced
*** Maximum pulse defined as 220 minus age in years

Make sure that you are training in the aerobic range, otherwise unhealthy levels of lactate (lactic acid salt) will be present in your body. This will not harm your baby but it can happen that your child does not like the taste of your milk due to the resulting acidity. Whenever possible, nurse before training. Around an hour after training, the concentration of lactic acid in your body will have normalized. If your baby has shorter nursing intervals, pump some milk ahead of time in preparation for an intensive training session.
Nursing before training also has the further positive effect that your breasts will feel empty and light and you will not feel any unpleasant tension there.

Supplementary workout

Gymnastic exercise after childbirth is aimed, above all, at strengthening the base of your pelvis. You can additionally perform the exercises for training during pregnancy (page 113). Begin at the very earliest in the fourth week after delivery with training for your pelvis and oblique abdominal muscles. You can start working on smooth abdominal muscles only in the fourth month after delivery, otherwise the opening of your smooth muscles will increase in size (rectus diastase).

Do not be too impatient! Your body has changed over the course of nine months. It needs almost as long to recuperate after this time.

Walking with baby

You can start walking with your newborn right away. Place your child in a suitable baby carriage and train very lightly in a kind of pre-walking: walk briskly and quickly over a period of at least 15 to 20 minutes.

The proper baby carriage

Starting at roughly the eighth or ninth month, when your child is able to sit, you can take it speed walking with you in a special carriage.
Even if the strain of the carriage while speed walking is less than it is when running, a so-called jogger or jogging carriage is optimal for walking. You should look out for a couple things in this case:

CAUTION: RISK OF INJURY!

IMPORTANT !

Your tendons, ligaments, and joints will be excessively soft and elastic for a few weeks after you give birth. For this reason you will be susceptible to a higher risk of accident.

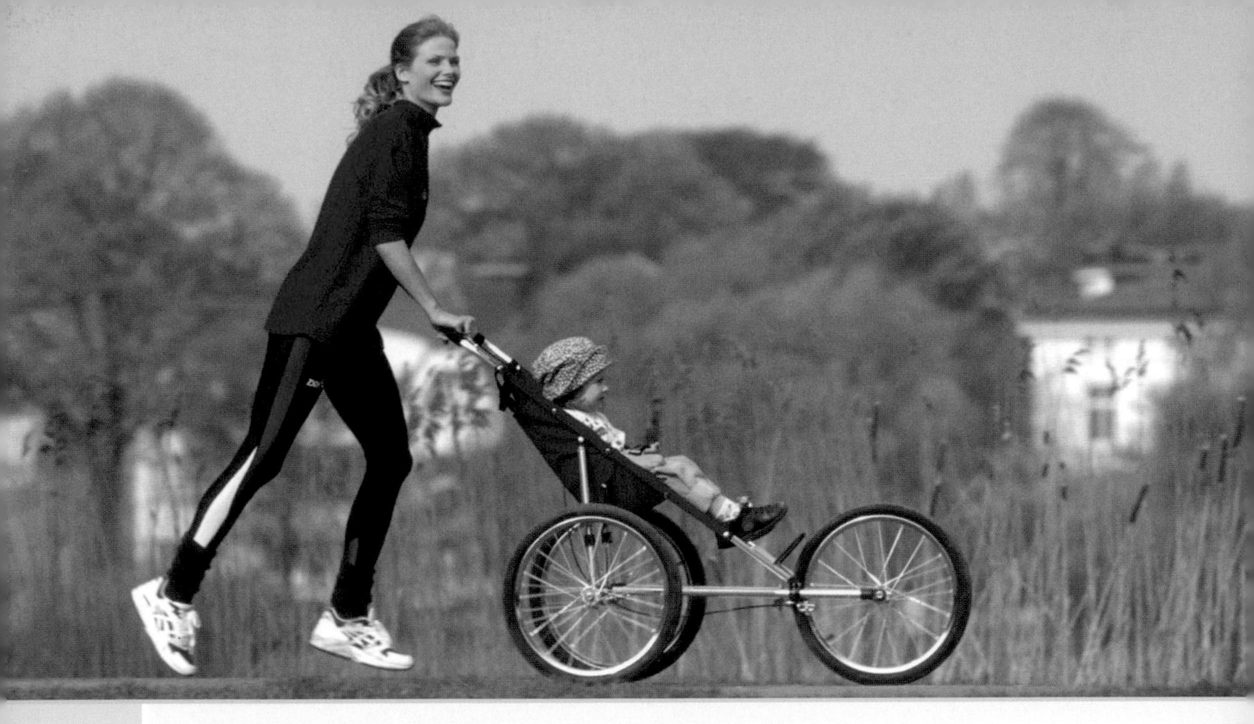

With the right “jogger” walking can be fun for mother and child.

- The safety of your child is of particular importance and is measured by a three- or, even better, five-star belt system, a high and stable side-guard, and a well-functioning handbrake. Sufficient protection from the sun (at least factor 30) should be taken into consideration. If you plan to walk at night with your child, visible reflectors are a must.
- Walking on field, forest, and meadow paths is more fun than on the street. Large air tires with good traction (or air chamber wheels that don’t have to be inflated) make speed walking easy even on uneven paths. They adapt to the terrain as well as to the child’s weight. Make sure before you buy a jogger that you won’t stub your toes on the connecting rod between the two rear wheels when walking.
- The better the shock absorbtion, the easier your training will be for your child, even on bumpy paths.
- If people of differing height plan to use the carriage, it’s a good idea to choose one with an adjustable handlebar. Hand straps will ensure that the walker always has the carriage under control – also when going downhill.
- Don’t forget a rain guard.

Index

Index of exercises

The most important points at a glance

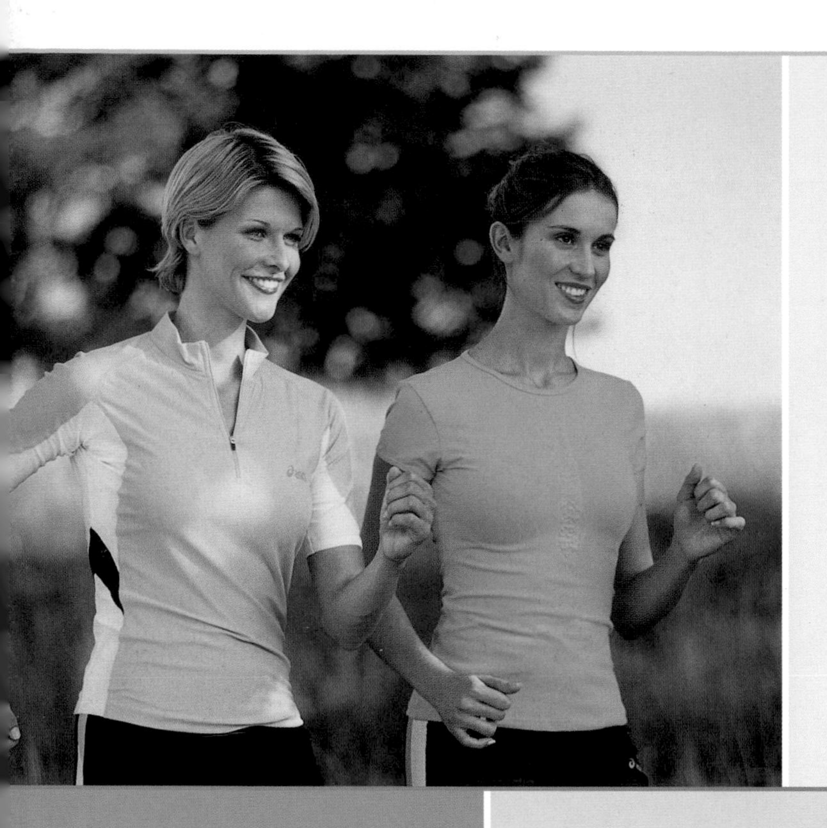

OVERCOMING STRESS

Speed walking in the open air can help you forget stress and the everyday problems at work and home. A great deal of endorphins, such as the creativity hormone ACTH, are released while walking. Your capacity for concentration and your attention span will be noticeably sharpened in the open air.

FATBURNER

The pounds slide away with speed walking! Your body burns plenty of calories when walking at a moderate pace, especially if you walk regularly. The fat burning effect is highest for regular speed walkers. Your body's basal metabolic rate rises as well. You use more energy – and not only while walking, but the whole day long.

SHOES AND CLOTHING

Walk only with well-fitting walking shoes. ou achieve your optimal motion range by continually working with your feet. An excellent shock absorbtion system is important to prevent damage to your joints and ligaments. Go for functional synthetic fibers in your choice of clothing. Breathable clothing functions as a warmth regulator: it prevents chill from evaporation and your skin remains dry and comfortably warm.

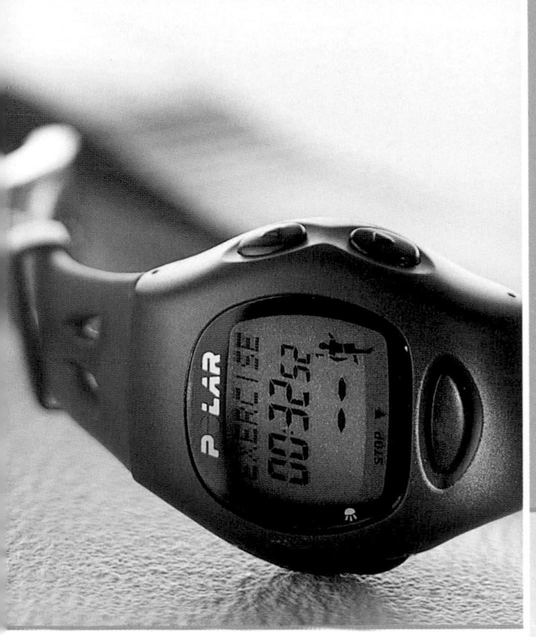

TAKING BREAKS

Speed walking has a healthy, invigorating effect only through a balance of exertion and relaxation. The reason is that your body supplies additional energy reserves, as a precaution, during regenerative periods of rest, which then enable higher stamina for your next training session. The result: your endurance increases.

NORDIC WALKING

The new walking trend is called Nordic walking. You speed walk with special walking sticks. These promote very active arm use and provide sufficient support in uneven terrain as well. Nordic walking is a healthy, full body sport in which your joints are less burdened than they are in "normal" speed walking. Also, the exertion of your arm muscles heightens energy use.
For this reason you burn around 40 percent more calories when Nordic walking.

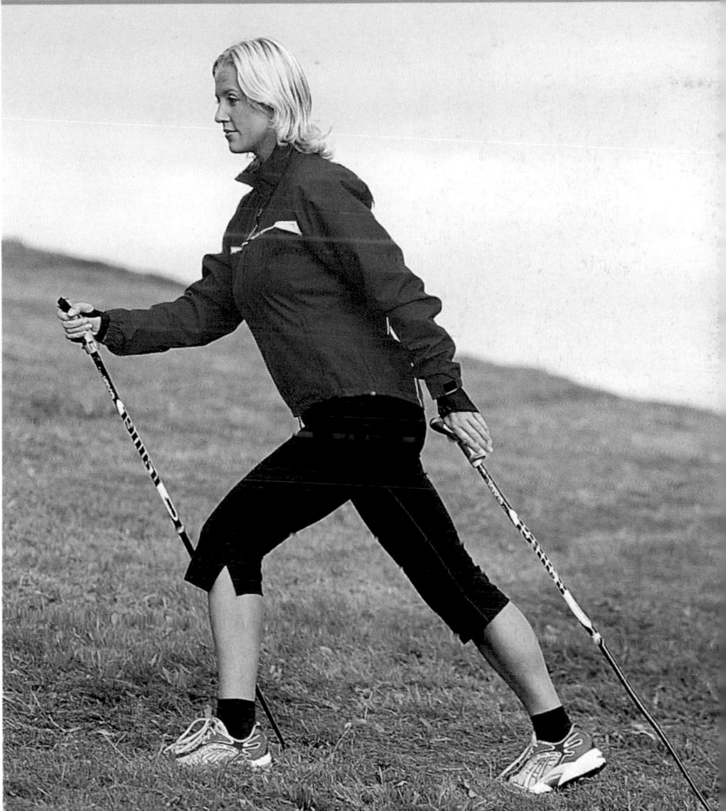

TRAINING PULSE

Pulse frequency is a good indicator of the intensity of physical activity. The more you exert yourself, the higher your pulse rises. You can determine your personal optimal training pulse rate with a simple formula: 220 heartbeats minus age in years will give you your maximum pulse (MP). Multiply this figure by 75 to 80 percent for heart and circulatory training. If you want to lose weight, multiply your MP by 60 to 70 percent (fat burning zone) and walk longer.

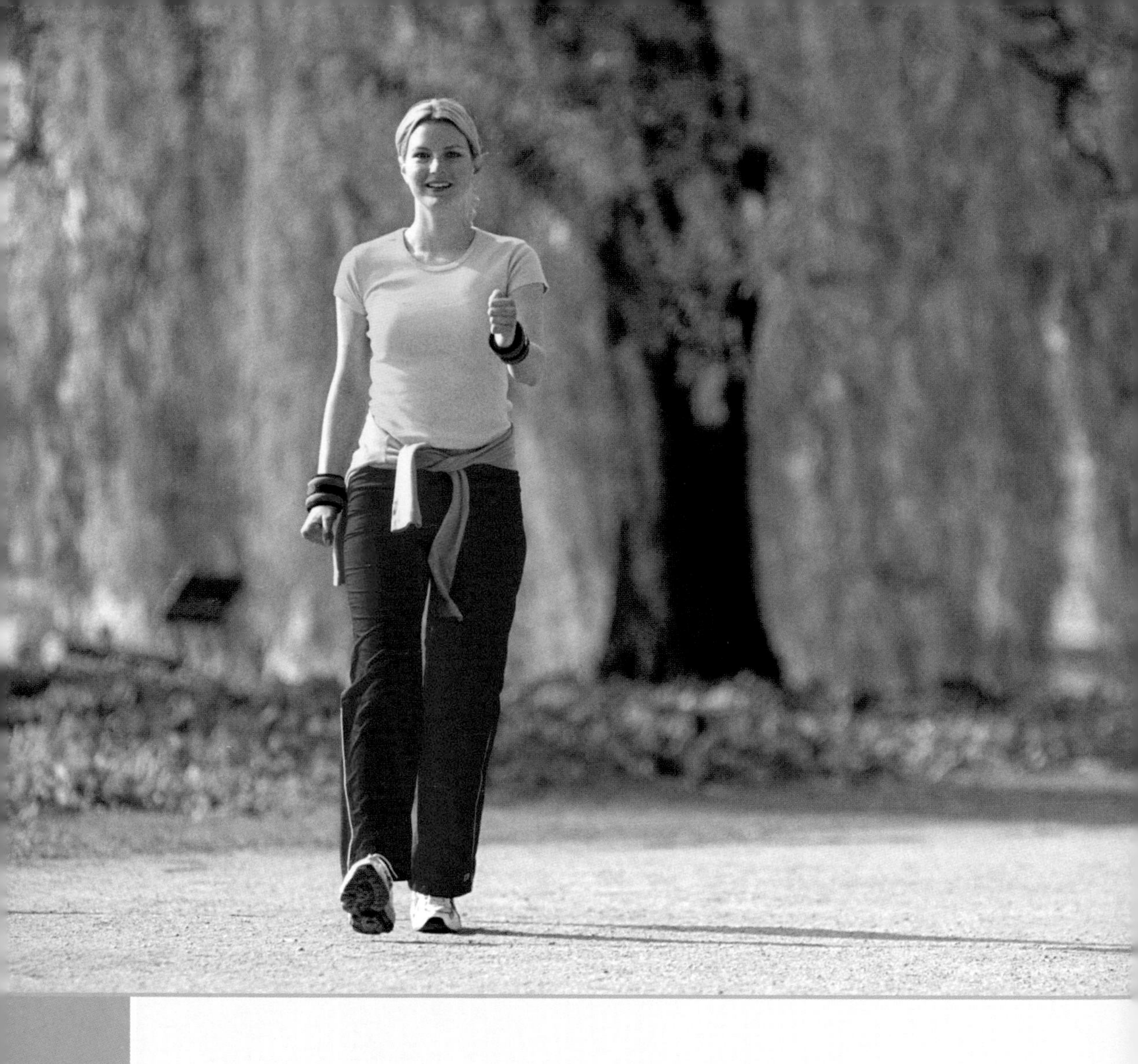

THE AUTHOR

Dr. Klaus Bös is Professor of Sports Science and head of the Institute for Sports and Sports Science at the University of Karlsruhe. In his research he deals with sports and health as well as with sports development, among other things. Speed walking is a particular highlight of his activities. Dr. Bös was one of the first to bring speed walking to Germany and founded the German Walking Institute, which he heads. The author has composed numerous technical publications and practical books about speed walking and fitness sports. He is scientific advisor to the German Gymnastic Federation and the German Athletic Association.